USE IT OR YOU'LL LOSE IT

USE IT OR, YOU'LL LOSE IT

Joseph Poticha, M.D.
with Art Southwood

RICHARD MAREK PUBLISHERS
NEW YORK

Copyright © 1978 by Joseph S. Poticha, M.D., and Art Southwood

All rights reserved. No part of this book may be reproduced in any form or by any means without prior written permission of the Publisher, excepting brief quotes used in connection with reviews written specifically for inclusion in a magazine or newspaper. For information write to Richard Marek Publishers, Inc., 200 Madison Avenue, New York, N.Y. 10016.

Library of Congress Cataloging in Publication Data

Poticha, Joseph S
Use it or you'll lose it.

Bibliography
Includes index
1. Sex instruction for the aged. I. Southwood, Art, joint author. II. Title.
HQ55.P68   613.9'5   78-13130
ISBN 0-399-90020-9

PRINTED IN THE UNITED STATES OF AMERICA

Second Impression

ACKNOWLEDGMENTS

Everyone who has touched my life contributed in some way to the realization of this book. To all of those family, friends, colleagues, and patients—who are, unfortunately, far too numerous to mention individually—my sincerest thanks.

There are some whom I would like to single out for special mention because of the specific help and encouragement they have given me:

•My niece, Sherry Narens, who found me both a publisher and a coauthor—and halfway through the book gave me a nephew when she married that coauthor. Thanks to her also for encouraging us when we needed it, and hollering at us, when that was called for.

•Dr. Bernard Shulman, Professor of Psychiatry at Loyola University School of Medicine, Chicago, and head of the Department of Psychiatry, St. Joseph's Hospital, Chicago, who first gave me the idea of writing a book.

•My two sons, Dr. Stuart Poticha, Associate Professor of Surgery, Northwestern University School of Medicine; and Dr. Gerald Poticha, Assistant Professor of Endocrinology, University of Colorado School of Medicine, for encouraging me when at times I felt like giving up. They also made many helpful suggestions from their own medical experiences.

•My dear friends, Peter and Ruth Tarrell, both social workers in geriatrics, who sponsored my first public lectures on sex for older people, and through whom I was invited to participate in the meetings of the National Council for the Aged in Chicago in 1973, which gained me international attention for my views.

•Another old and dear friend, Harry Lowitz, who gave me much encouragement, and some valuable insights from his point of view as a layman.

•My nurse-assistant Laurel Fishman and my office secretary Geraldine Simon, who cheerfully took on many, many hours of extra work to help me complete this book.

•My agent, Dominick Abel, whose faith in the book finally overcame the many obstacles to achieving publication.

•And last, but not least, Joyce Engelson, Editor-in-Chief of Richard Marek Publishers, whose sharp eye, practical criticisms, and unflagging enthusiasm brought the project to a successful conclusion.

To Helen and Joan, the two women in my life.

CONTENTS

	Preface	11
1	Sex—What Has Age Got to Do with It?	15
2	Your Sex Organs	28
3	How Your Sex Organs Work	39
4	Why You Men Might Think You're Impotent	50
5	Frigidity and Why Women Fail to Respond Sexually	64
6	Men and Masturbation	79
7	Women and Masturbation	89
8	Achieving Sexual Satisfaction	98
9	What If You've Been Sick?	110
10	What If You've Had an Operation?	122
11	Having (and Being) an Interesting and Interested Partner	131
12	Specific Male Problems	143
13	Specific Female Problems	154
14	Sexually Transmitted Diseases	164
15	Getting Back into the Swing of Things	172
16	The Attitudes of Others, and Some Odds and Ends	183
	Seeking Professional Help	191
	Suggestions for Further Reading	193
	Index	197

PREFACE

One of the biggest surprises I got in my early years as a doctor was the discovery that people in their sixties, seventies, even eighties and beyond, could continue to have sex. You can be sure it was a pleasant surprise. I enjoyed sex, and the prospect of being able to have it virtually all my life was a happy one.

Thanks to the research that has been done in recent years on human sexuality, the idea of sex for senior citizens is nowhere near as mind-boggling as it was in the old days. But I can tell you from my own experiences as a doctor and a lecturer—the possibility of sex at any age much over fifty catches an awful lot of people by surprise. As in my case, the surprise is usually a pleasant one. Time and again I have seen my audience light up the lecture hall with their joy when I have told them they need not give up the pleasures of physical love, just because they are older.

Sex researchers might know a good deal nowadays about sex for the elderly, but from what I can see, the information isn't getting to the people. And there's no doubt in my mind the people want that information. The reactions I get from my talks, and the letters I receive in response to newspaper interviews and appearances on talk shows are proof to me of that. What's more, a question I could always count on hearing from a good many people after a lecture was, "Where can I get a copy of your book?" For many years I had to say, "I'm afraid I haven't written a book." To which the usual reply has been, "Well, then, why don't you?" So now I have.

I've tried to keep the presentation casual and straightforward and not weigh you down with reams of information and statistics that are primarily of interest to doctors and sex researchers. Although there are some limits to what can be done in the pages of a book, I've tried to give you the same kind of help and guidance you would get if you consulted me in person. However, if what you read here gives you a thirst for more specialized or scholarly information, you'll find suggestions for further reading at the end of the book.

The book is as much a practical workbook as I could make it. If I haven't stressed the romantic, hearts-and-flowers aspects of sex, believe me, it's not because I don't think those things are important. But there are many, many other books which deal with those things. Anyway, romance is really magic, isn't it? Magic is different for everybody. How can I possibly tell you what is going to make magic happen for you? I can't! All I can say is, when it happens, go with it. That's why I'm sticking to the things I can tell you that are likely to do you some practical good.

Who is this book for? I think I can say it's for almost everybody past the age of twenty-five. No, I'm not kidding. Sure, most of the attention is given to the problems of older people—people in their fifties, sixties and over. Just remember this—many of those problems start years before a person ever reaches fifty or sixty. There is much of value here for younger readers—if nothing else, the knowledge that in many ways the best part of their sexual lives is still ahead of them. So much for age. What about marital status? It doesn't matter. I've tried to take into account the problems of married couples, of unmarried couples, and of single men and women without regular sex partners.

Writing about sex is tricky at best, and sometimes the line between frankness and coarseness is a thin one. I've tried not to cross that line, and I think I've succeeded. However, I realize that even the most well-intentioned frankness can be disturbing to some readers. Some of you will be bothered by ideas and suggestions that are contrary to things you have been taught to believe. Many sexually oriented books carry a warning to the effect that if frankness offends you, stay away. I won't say that. In fact, I'll tell you just the opposite. If something you read in this book disturbs you or even offends you, please bear with me. Remember, I'm speaking to you as a doctor, and I'm telling you exactly what I would tell you if I were seeing you privately in my office. Please keep in mind that somehing you might accept quite calmly if I told it to you in person can look mighty startling if you see it in print. I'm out to help you, not shock you, after all.

There's one last thing you might like to know about me in connection with the theme of this book. At this writing I'm seventy years of age—and I practice what I preach!

Joseph S. Poticha, M.D.

Chapter 1:
SEX—WHAT HAS AGE GOT TO DO WITH IT?

Suppose somebody told you that you shouldn't read books or magazines anymore, you shouldn't kiss the people you love, you shouldn't even visit with your friends—because you're "too old." You'd probably hit the ceiling. "Why, that's preposterous!" you'd say. "I have a right to do those things. What's my age got to do with it?"

Exactly! What has your age got to do with it? You have a right to fulfill yourself mentally, emotionally, and socially. You have that right no matter what your age. But you have another right you may have forgotten about or let yourself be talked out of. You have a right to fulfill yourself *sexually*. In fact, you not only have the right to fulfill yourself sexually, you probably have the ability to do it, too.

"Well," you might say, "that's a nice theory, but it probably wouldn't work for me." That's exactly the kind of attitude I've spent much of my professional life fighting, and it's the big reason for writing this book. If you say, "it won't work," my response is, why not? What makes you so special, so different from other people your age that you think you can't have sex?

Right now, before you read another word, stop and make a list of ten reasons why you think it wouldn't work for you. Without seeing the list or knowing anything about you but the fact that you're reading this book, it's pretty safe for me to say that at least seven of those reasons are pure nonsense—and the other three can probably be overcome with a little effort on your part.

I saw a bumper sticker recently that said, "old gymnasts never die—they just can't remount in 30 seconds." That's how it is with sex. What used to happen fast when you were younger now happens slower. *But it still happens!* Yes, sex in the later years is possible. It's important for you to understand that when I say "later years" I don't mean forty-three or forty-four, I mean after seventy, and even after eighty—as long as you keep it up and don't quit. The phrase "use it or you'll lose it" is true, but even if you have lost it, you can probably get it back.

Maybe you find that hard to believe. But one thing is certain—you want to believe it. You wouldn't be reading this book if you didn't. However, I have been making some pretty bold statements, and I can't blame you if you want to see me back them up with some proof.

For starters, I could give you the names of several senior citizens whose names are household words who have proved their sexual potency in the most definite way possible—by fathering children at an age when most people assumed they were already out to pasture. One who leaps to mind is the late Bing Crosby, who started an entire second family at an age when many men have given up sexually. However, far better proof can be seen in the large numbers of my own patients in their seventies and eighties who are still having regular intercourse—and enjoying it.

Many of those patients of mine were like many of you. They had lost their sexual ability, and they were afraid it was gone forever. But they have been helped to regain that lost sexual ability, and very likely you can be, too.

Another solid block of evidence comes from the world of scientific research, going all the way back to Kinsey. In more recent years Masters and Johnson and many others have discussed the subject of sex for older people in their books and have compiled extensive statistics on the sexual potency of older people.

If you were to wade through all the research on human sexuality from Kinsey on, you'd run across some interesting statistics: four out of five men in their sixties and older are interested in sex. Sixty-five percent of men in their sixties are doing something about it. And so are 25 percent of men in their seventies and older.

The numbers are a little lower for women. Thirty-three percent of women in their sixties report continued sexual activities. Do you wonder why women are less active sexually? Part of the reason is a lack of available partners for older women. However, studies have shown us one major reason: when both husband and wife stop having sex, 86 percent of the time it is the husband's responsibility. That's one statistic I hope this book can help change!

Those numbers are impressive, but the most impressive fact to come out of all that research into sexuality is—*there is no single age you can point to when people actually stop having intercourse.*

I have to admit, though, there was a time when I thought sex for older people was highly improbable. In fact, when I was a medical student, there wasn't one person in my class who wouldn't have gladly settled for a *life span* of sixty-five. If we weren't counting on living much past middle age, we sure weren't counting on having sex that long! In those days it was a very common idea that men went through a change of life just as women did. But we didn't know that the change of life in women made no change in their sexual appetites. We assumed their sexual needs did change—and naturally we assumed the same for men. But while I was an intern in King County Hospital in Seattle in the early thirties, I had an experience that gave me quite a jolt.

I used to be on call at a clinic the hospital operated in the red-light district. One day an eighty-two-year-old man came into the clinic with gonorrhea. I was dumbfounded when I saw him. I said to him, "Grandpa, where'd you get this?" And he snorted, "Where do you suppose I got it?" He was fit to be tied. He came down once a month from the mountains. He'd gone to the same house for more than thirty years, and he never got a dose. This time he got a dose, and he was madder than hell. The old guy was plenty spry, too. There is only one way he could have gotten gonorrhea, so he was telling the truth.

As I said, the experience gave me—and everybody connected with the clinic—quite a jolt. Here was a man almost twenty years past what we considered to be a normal life span, and he was still having sex. He was more than unusual—he was a phenomenon!

I thought he was a fluke at the time, but over the years I have seen a good deal of evidence that he wasn't a fluke at all. Don't forget, this all happened a good forty-five years ago. In those days older folks didn't talk about what they did sexually, because in those days it was considered wrong. All too many people still cling to that outmoded attitude, but that's something I want to talk about later.

In the early days of my medical practice, none of the sexual data we now take for granted had been collected yet and no studies of sexuality were available, so I had to learn about it gradually from my own patients. And, of course, my attitudes on sexuality were guided by what I was learning. At first I wasn't trying to help my patients with their sexual problems. I was simply trying to find out what was going on. Fortunately, my attitude toward sex was a healthy one. I wasn't afraid to ask my patients about it; I was willing to learn and I wasn't embarrassed by their stories. I began to be able to apply what I was learning from one patient to the problems of other patients.

At first my questions about sex were mere curiosity. To my surprise, the more I investigated, the more I came across instances of people continuing sexual activity well past the age I had been taught all such things stopped. I began to realize that sexuality was an important part of human living, and that it didn't necessarily stop just because of age. That was a very encouraging and comforting discovery.

One of my early patients was a woman in her forties who had just married a man in his middle sixties. I was curious enough to ask her what sort of sex life she was leading. I thought her medical problem might have had something to do with her sex life, because she was a young woman who was probably still sexually vigorous married to a man I was sure was too old to function successfully. I had a feeling that some of her symptoms were from frustration. So I asked her, "Do you have any kind of sex life at all? Is John any good?" To my utter astonishment, she told me they had intercourse at least three times a week, and he was very effective. Much more effective than her first husband.

I was very much surprised at the time, mostly out of ignorance and inexperience. However, over the years I have found that what happened to her is a common thing. Many women who have had poor sexual experiences in a first marriage find a second marriage much more invigorating and much more satisfying sexually. The same is true for men, of course.

Another patient I remember vividly was a woman in her late forties married to a man in his seventies. I was treating her for a pelvic infection, and I happened to remark on how lucky she was not to have to worry about sexual intercourse aggravating her condition. "I wish you would tell that to my husband," she said. "That man bothers me each and every night." It turned out that one of the reasons she married him was she had never cared too much about sex and thought a man of his age wouldn't care too much about it, either. She even told him she wished he would find one or two other women to get his pleasure from so he would leave her alone.

You know, that's exactly what he did! The reason I know about it is he introduced me to two of his girlfriends—young women he was having relations with. He was seventy-five at the time, but he was plenty potent, and the girlfriends were happy to attest to it.

As a result of those experiences—and many more like them—I became a believer. I even had an opportunity to see at first hand how wrong my earlier attitudes were, when my first wife died. I was already in my sixties then.

When it happened, the shock was a great one. It didn't help much at all being a doctor and knowing exactly what was wrong and how inevitable it all was. Just like everybody else, I was completely unprepared. I found out very quickly how dependent I was on her. I was a doctor; I attended to my own profession and she took care of everything else. So when she died, the bottom fell out. I felt totally helpless.

I didn't even know how to boil a kettle of water. So at first I allowed myself to be enveloped by my dear friends and my brother and sisters. They helped me as much as they could, but I was still coming back to a lonely home with lots of memories, and that only increased my depression. After the initial grief was past, I went into another stage. I began to feel that I was imposing on people and that things were being done for me because people felt sorry for me. I felt like a fifth wheel. During that whole time the thought of sex never occurred to me.

Of course, as my wife's illness had progressed, sex had become less and less frequent, and had finally stopped altogether when it became something she wasn't able to handle. I suppose by the time I started to withdraw from my friends, I was as typical a case of lost sexual potency as I had ever treated in my own practice.

When I got to the point where I completely lost interest in my work, I did one of the smartest things I've ever done for myself in my life—I went into therapy. It took a while, but that turned things around for me, and gradually I began to emerge socially again, and even began to date. The women I went out with at that time were all women I knew or women who were introduced to me by friends whose judgment I trusted. In most instances the women were in their fifties or older. Oh, sure, I was attracted to younger women, but I knew I would rather go out with women who were closer to the age of a woman I might be interested in marrying.

Most of the women I dated were widows, and I was amazed at the intense, pent-up emotions these women had, how much excitement and sexual drive they had. Although my drive in the beginning was down to nothing, I found myself attempting sex, and my drive began to return. Because my sex life had been vigorous when I was young, it wasn't long before I became vigorous again. One of my greatest pleasures at that time was the discovery that I was able to find an active sex life with older women and I didn't have to start running around with twenty-year-olds.

It pleased me to discover in my own experience that women

never lose their sexual powers and can maintain their vigor indefinitely. I don't mind telling you I was also highly gratified to be able to see in myself that the things I had been reading and telling my patients about restoring sexual vigor in men were true. What it comes down to, you see, is that I'm not trying to sell you a lot of fancy theory that won't stand up. I know it isn't just theory, because I went through it myself.

So here's something else for you to believe. Sex in the later years is not only possible, it's possible for *you*. What's more, a good sex life can do a lot to make you a healthy, attractive, vital person. I've been aware for a long time that older men and women who have an active sex life look and feel better than other people in their age group. Now I'm not saying that sex is the only thing that does it, but there is no doubt that sexual activity is a very healthy thing. Not only that; a person who has kept himself or herself interested and active sexually isn't about to give up enjoying life's other pleasures. One thing leads to another, and you're sure to find sexually active people on the golf courses, in the swimming pools, involved with creative hobbies, ceramics, crafts, painting, and so on—in short, keeping active, because they are alive and vital and interested in life.

On the other hand, I've had older people come to me and say, "I'm exhausted." "I can't eat." "I have pains." "I don't feel good." Much of the time a careful examination reveals there's nothing wrong with them physically at all. They're depressed. They may not sit at home and cry all the time, but they're depressed. The thought of aging is a common cause of depression in both men and women. Men realize they are no longer the "studs" they once were. They see themselves getting older and past their prime. Women feel they are losing their feminine charms and are no longer attractive. The loss of a loved one can cause a very serious depression. But give those same people a romance, and suddenly they perk up. I've seen it happen time and again. Romance is the best cure I know for depression.

Let me give you an example. I had a patient with diabetes who had always managed to keep herself in good health and her illness well under control. She had no children, and she was deeply involved with her husband. Then he died suddenly, and she went into a severe depression. I tried to keep in touch with her because I was afraid of what might happen to her health. My fears were well-founded. As a result of her depression, her diabetes went completely out of control, because she disregarded her medications and became extremely careless about what she ate. In fact, she only ate when she was forced to.

Over the next couple of years she was constantly in and out of hospitals as I fought a losing battle to control her diabetes. I even sent her to psychotherapy, because of the seriousness of her depression, which I wasn't qualified to treat.

For a long time, nothing seemed to work. Then one day when she came to my office, she seemed to be looking a little better. Not a lot better, but at least better. She was a little more cheerful. Her blood sugar was beginning to improve, and when I questioned her about her diet, I found she was eating more regularly. In fact, she had begun to put on a little weight.

After the improvement continued in a second and then a third visit, I finally said, "Janet, tell me what happened to make you suddenly become a good patient again." She hemmed and she hawed and she blushed, but she finally said, "Well, doctor, you won't believe this, but a very old friend of the family who I've always sort of secretly admired came to visit me one day and began to show a lot of interest in me. We talked a lot at first, and he told me the same things you have told me and that the psychiatrist has told me, but it seemed different coming from him. He made me feel special enough that I wanted to do what he asked me to do."

The friendship continued to develop, she said, and then, "As soon as I felt well enough, we started dating. I can't tell you, doctor, how quickly my whole life started to look better to me and how much better I'm beginning to feel." A little more questioning on my part revealed that they were getting sexually involved with each other and were talking quite seriously about marriage. When she left my office that time, she said, "You're not going to be bothered with me being sick much longer. You'll find me just the kind of patient I was before."

And that's just what happened. She began to dress better, she began to use makeup, and every time I saw her she looked more attractive. There's nothing magic about it, though. One of the things an active sex life does is give you an incentive to keep yourself attractive. It makes you more careful about how you dress and take care of yourself. You want to look as good as you feel.

Another thing it does is keep you open to other people. You don't lose touch with the real joy human contact can give. You don't dry up inside. It's got to make you feel great to realize you haven't had to give up an important part of your life just because you're older. With all that going for you, it's pretty hard to feel depressed!

But maybe it's been a while since you've been active sexually, and getting started again seems like a pretty tall order.

For most people, sex means intercourse—erection, penetration, and orgasm for the man, and an orgasm for the woman. That's how it is for young people. In most cases, it can be that way for you, too. But it isn't even necessary to have "penis-in-vagina" sex to enjoy it. There are many other ways for you to get full pleasure from sexual contact.

Sex for you could be something simpler. You don't always have to make it a bedtime relationship. It can be the warmth and the closeness of companionship, security, someone to talk to, someone to communicate with, someone to feel near you at night when you wake up from a bad dream. And most important, it can mean someone to love and care for.

I had a patient who had a stroke and was totally incapable of "penis-in-vagina" sex. He has to wear a catheter because he can't control his urine. He and his wife sleep in separate beds. Do they have a sexual relationship? You bet they do! As his wife told me, "Just the fact that I can cuddle up to him and he can feel me near him gives me a feeling of warmth and satisfaction. I even feel excited sexually, though he's paralyzed and can't touch me."

Feeling relaxed about sex isn't always easy, because there's so much emphasis put on performance these days. Just remember, there's a lot of pleasure in simply touching, manipulating, and fondling—all of which are forms of sexual expression. If you're having trouble getting started, you'll find that fondling, touching, kissing, and getting reacquainted with each other physically often does reawaken sexual desire.

Sometimes a playful mood can suddenly bring forth an erection that hasn't been there for a long time. Don't get discouraged if an erection happens and then softens right away when you try to use it. If you had an erection at all—no matter how brief—that means it's still possible for you. And each time is going to get better.

It's going to be better for you women, too. With the longer period of fondling and touching, suppressed or dormant sexual feelings will suddenly be reawakened to excitement. That's going to make sex much more satisfying for you, and in many instances it will give you time to have an orgasm.

I had a patient come to me recently, a woman of seventy-five. She had read a newspaper article on a talk I gave about sex for older people. She's a fine-looking woman, and you wouldn't take her for more than fifty-five or sixty. She must have been a killer when she was younger. She had been widowed for twenty years, and she admitted to me that she'd never had an orgasm in her entire life. By the time I saw her, she was very uninterested in sex. It didn't mean much to her.

She was attractive enough so she had plenty of dates. I never asked her if she went to bed with any of them. She obviously did a few times and never got anything out of it, so she figured sex was a big nothing as far as she was concerned. Then she met a man in his late seventies who wined her, dined her, courted her, and finally bedded her. She had the first orgasm of her life with him. What made the difference? Well, from the conversation I had with her, the biggest factor was his age. He could still have sex, but it took him a while. That extra time turned out to be all she needed to bring her to the pitch of excitement she needed to have an orgasm.

Their relationship has developed into a wonderful, satisfying thing for both of them, and the last I heard, they were planning to get married.

She's one of the best proofs I've ever seen that a person in good physical health with a willing and stimulating partner *is* capable of sex—at any age.

By the way, when I say "good health," I don't mean you have to be the Bionic Oldster to be able to have sex. No, I'm talking about an individual who has a reasonably good heart, walks four or more blocks a day without getting short of breath, and is able to perform his or her usual daily chores.

So if you think you have to be able to jog five miles a day or swim fifty laps of the pool, or play three sets of tennis or a couple of rounds of golf a day—stop worrying. That's not what I mean at all. Basically, I'm talking about an ordinary man or woman in their sixties or seventies or older who lives a relatively normal life, perhaps goes to work regularly and enjoys going out to dinner and the theatre once in a while. If you're a woman and you can still maintain a household, that's healthy enough, as far as I'm concerned.

Many of you have had an illness such as a stroke, or arthritis, or have recovered from heart attacks and are now capable of living normal lives. That's the kind of good health I'm talking about. If you have been ill, there are ways you can tell if you have recovered enough for sex, and we'll go into all that later. Right now, though, I just want to assure you that you haven't been thrown out of the game for life.

Maybe by now you're beginning to believe you *can* have sex at your age, but you can't make yourself believe you should. This is a good place to make an important point: too many people are foolishly denying themselves the joy of sexual pleasure because they fear being called a "dirty old man" or "silly old lady." It's a sad thing indeed when so many people believe behavior that's perfectly acceptable when you are young somehow gets foolish when you are older.

It's hard to avoid those negative attitudes. No matter where you go, somebody seems to be ready with a snide remark. It's hard to stay calm in the face of a remark one widow told me her children made when she came home late from a date— "Don't tell me you're shacking up with him!"

I know of other people—widows and widowers both—who have suffered the embarrassment of seeing their children treat their dates with outright rudeness and hostility.

My profession brings me into nursing homes from time to time, and I can't begin to keep track of how many times nurses and other staff members in those homes have complained to me about how much trouble they have keeping the men and women from going into each other's rooms. They usually add a remark something like, "Can you imagine those old folks trying to get sexy?"

You can hardly turn on television anymore without seeing some comedian making snide remarks and poking fun at the idea of older people having sex.

And last but not least, you can't escape the attitudes of your peers. All too often, the worst bad-mouthing of sex for older people comes from folks our age. For this one I don't have to give you any examples—just listen the next time you get together with your friends. That situation reminds me of a famous line uttered by the comic-strip character, Pogo: "We have met the enemy, and he is us!"

Attitudes are changing, because longer life spans mean more older people are around than ever before. But those attitudes are a long way from being changed completely. You're still going to have to buck those attitudes, and it's going to take a certain amount of courage. Just remember—you have a *right* to enjoy sex. You've got to really believe you have that right. Only if you believe in it, will what follows in this book have any meaning for you—or have any chance of success.

But once it starts working, you won't worry much about feeling foolish—you'll be too busy feeling good!

If you're willing to take the plunge, you can be a part of something you've only been reading about for the past few years—the sexual revolution. That's not as farfetched as it might sound. The idea of sex in the later years is turning out to be a lot more revolutionary than some of the things those young people have been thinking up. When you get right down to it, it's about time the older people joined the revolution.

You're going to have to do some educating, though. You're going to have to educate yourself, first of all, and rid yourself of those myths and bugaboos that are standing in your way. You're going to have to educate your children and other young people to realize that you are still able to have sex. You'll have to help them understand that just because you might be a grandparent, the bedroom isn't lost to you.

Much has to be done to educate the people who deal with the elderly. That means everybody from social workers to the folks who run nursing homes. They've got to be made to realize how wrong it is to have such things as separate floors for the men and women. They've got to be convinced of the importance of such things as a quiet room with a TV set and a couch, and enough privacy so people can cuddle a little if they want to.

Am I asking you to take on those institutions single-handed? Certainly not. There are many organizations of older people doing that work already. One or more of them is probably operating in your community. The way you could help would be to give them whatever support you can—be it financial, emotional, or volunteering to stuff envelopes.

Between the sexual revolution and the women's liberation movement, more people are challenging values and ideas than ever before. You couldn't have picked a better time to start. You already have started, you know. Just by reading this far, you've asked yourself a very important question— "Why not me?"

The answer to that question is what this book is all about. I'm going to put to rest the myths and groundless fears that sex in the later years is either wrong or unlikely. I'll also show you how to deal with the changes that might occur in your body because of age—changes that could complicate the usual ways of functioning sexually. I'll be talking about things like your feelings about yourself and the opposite sex, the problems of physical limitations, and coping with the attitudes of other (especially younger) people toward your sex life.

If you haven't been active sexually for a while, you've probably forgotten just how your body works. So the first thing I'll talk about is your sex organs.

Chapter 2:
YOUR SEX ORGANS

Remember the old story about the Frenchman who overheard someone remark that men and women are different? He ran down the street shouting, *"Vive la différence!"* Yes, you men and women are different from each other physically, but you've got a lot more in common than you think, especially where your sex organs are concerned.

Would it surprise you to know that for almost the first three months in the womb the sex organs of both male and female are exactly the same? That's right, exactly the same. In fact, they look like the female organ. Sometime between the tenth and the twelfth week, a whole series of amazing changes begins to take place and nature starts to separate the boys from the girls.

How does the embryo become either male or female? (An "embryo," by the way, is a developing baby in the first weeks within the womb; the next stage of development is called the "fetus.") As soon as the male sperm—which carries the gene that determines the sex of the child—unites with the ovum, the sex is already determined. Men, therefore, are entirely responsible for the sex of their children. That's pretty ironic when you think about it, because a lot of men have some funny ideas about how sex is determined.

One of my patients is a good example of that. When Sam's wife got pregnant, he did everything he could think of to make sure it was a boy. He told his wife, "I want a boy," as if he were ordering from a catalog. He wore every good-luck charm he could lay his hands on. He carried garlic in his pocket. After he ran through all his own superstitions, he began to ask his friends for *their* favorites. The upshot of that case is, Sam is very happy with his baby girl—but it took me a long time to convince him that he had already sired a daughter long before he even began all the mumbo-jumbo. So if any of you men have secretly or openly blamed your wives for all your children being the same sex, or if any of you women have had a sense of guilt about it—now you know who's responsible.

Before the changes, the sex organ looks like a bulb with a groove below it and a swelling on either side. Then at the top of the bulb, a small nubbin appears. A hormone is secreted which starts either the masculinizing changes which make the external sex organs male, or the feminizing changes which make them female. The particular hormone which masculinizes is testosterone, and the one which feminizes is estrogen. The nubbin grows into a penis in the male, and in the female the nubbin becomes the clitoris.

The groove closes in the male to form a tube—the shaft of the penis. In females, this groove stays open and becomes the inner, or smaller, lips (labia minora) of the vagina. In females, the two swellings at the sides stay in place to form the outer lips (labia majora) of the vagina; in males, they drop down and fuse to become the scrotum, or sac. In both sexes, the sexual glands originate in the back of the abdomen. In the male, these glands (testicles) drop into the newly formed scrotum. The female sexual glands (ovaries) only descend as far as the pelvis or lower abdomen.

By the time a baby is born, all the necessary changes and shifts are finished, and everything is complete and in its proper place.

You may be wondering why I'm taking the trouble to tell you how your sexual development begins, and why a chapter on your sex organs is even necessary. After all, you've been walking around in that body of yours for quite some time now, and you should know what it looks like and how it works. Well, if you're like most people, you probably take your body pretty much for granted. When you were younger—especially as you went through puberty to adulthood—you were a lot more aware of your body and the changes that took place as you grew and developed into a sexual being.

As you got older, your body settled into maturity, and except for bouts with illness and disease, you became less aware of yourself physically. And, of course, you had other things to think about. Things like your job, your family, and community activities, for example. Or maybe you just didn't want to face the changes that happen naturally with aging. So you turned your attention to other things and simply forgot much of what you had learned about your physical self.

In all my years as a doctor, one thing has never ceased to astonish me—how little people actually know about their sex organs and how they work. I might add that it's more true of women than it is of men. After I became aware of this lack of knowledge in my patients, I began to throw in a little teaching with my examinations. For example, when I do a pelvic examination now, I like to use a mirror to show the woman what the inside of her vagina looks like and let her see the cervix, or mouth of the womb. I like to point out how small the cervix is, and how much it has to stretch to permit a baby to come out. I'm always careful at this point to explain that it is a painless area. There are no nerve endings in the cervix. This is all new information to most of these women!

You'd be amazed at the number of women who don't know where the clitoris is—and that's the most highly sensitive of all the female genital organs. Many women are surprised when I show them the opening of the urethra, through which they urinate. What surprises them? The fact that it's a separate opening from the vagina. A lot of women have never used tampons, and have never found out they don't urinate from the vagina.

It's been my experience that there is very little men don't know about their sex organs—everything is right out in the open where it can be seen. Another reason a man is more likely to be familiar with his sex organs is that he handles them a lot. He usually holds his penis to urinate, and he also touches his organs when he washes them in the bath or shower. A woman doesn't have those advantages. By the way, men don't know very much about women's sex organs, either.

I've noticed that this lack of knowledge shows up in the young people I treat, too. The way sex is talked about and written about so openly these days, that's amazing! From what I've seen, the youngsters of today talk a good game, but they don't really understand what they're talking about. At least you older folks have some excuse if you don't know too much about your sex organs and how they work. When you were young, sex was something that wasn't talked about much at all. If it was talked about, it was in whispers.

And don't forget, nobody really knew very much about the actual physiology of sex in those days, odd as that may seem. While a great deal has been written on sexuality in recent years, it was not until Kinsey's papers were published out of Indiana University, followed by the studies of Dr. Eric Pfeiffer and his colleagues at Duke University, Dr. Harold Lief's work at the University of Pennsylvania, and last of all the magnificent contributions of Masters and Johnson that we began to understand a little bit about sexuality in the elderly. Since then, many others too numerous to mention have added to our knowledge.

So if your background was governed by Victorian attitudes and hampered by a lack of information, you might have a lot to learn. Or maybe you did know your body pretty well when you were younger, but you haven't kept up with the changes that took place as you got older. Then what you need is a refresher course.

If you want to be effective sexually at *any* age, it's important for you to know what your sex organs are and how to use them. And now that you're older, you've also got to be aware of the changes that have come with age—in both you and your sex partner. Being aware of the changes is very important, because it can affect the way you function sexually.

You see your sex organs every day. But when was the last

time you *looked* at them? I mean really looked at them carefully. Maybe you feel shy or embarrassed about them. Some people seem to wish they didn't have sex organs at all, and that's nonsense. Your sex organs are every bit as natural a part of your body as your hands, your feet, or your nose. Your body was planned to have sex organs. You wouldn't be a completely formed human being without them.

Let's take a good look at each of the sex organs, starting with those of the woman. First I'll tell you what they are like in a younger woman, and then what happens with age, so you can understand the changes better.

One more thing before we start. If you're a man, don't skip the part about women, and if you're a woman, don't skip the part about men. The more you know about what makes your partner tick, the more effective you'll be as a partner.

Here's an example of what knowing your partner's body can mean. I told a man recently about how a woman's clitoris draws back completely into the skin that covers it when she reaches a certain state of arousal. Before I told him that, he had always wondered why he suddenly "lost" the clitoris while he was stimulating his sex partner. That led him to a lot of frantic fumbling around, and whatever pleasure she got was by sheer accident. But once he knew what was happening to her, he knew exactly where to find the clitoris. She told him afterward, "I've never been so excited in my life!"

Okay, now let's go.

The first thing you see is the pubic hair, which is usually shaped like an upside-down triangle. However, some women have pubic hair that comes up the belly to the navel. This bothers many of these women, but I don't know why it should. One of my patients has hair like that—a thin line from the top of the pubic thatch to her navel. She won't wear a two-piece swimsuit because of it, though she tells me her husband loves it. He thinks it's very sexy. Different people have different attitudes about body hair. Many European women, for example, don't understand why women in the United States insist on shaving underarm hair.

For most men and women, the pubic hair is the sum total of

what a vagina looks like. But this hair only covers the two outer lips, or labia majora. If you spread the outer lips, you'll see the two inner lips, or labia minora. The inner lips don't have hair on them, and they vary in color from pink to brown, depending on the woman's natural skin color. If a woman has had one or more pregnancies, the inner lips tend to be darker. This external part of the female sex organs is called the vulva.

One thing I'd like you all to be aware of—there is no such thing as a "standard" size or shape for the labia. They are shaped differently and are of different size from one woman to another. Why am I making a point of telling you this? Because it's something a lot of women really worry about. I've had women actually tell me they were ashamed because their labia were different from what they considered to be the norm.

Nancy is an example of that kind of unfortunate thinking. She had come to me for a checkup before joining a racquetball club. When I saw her again several months later, I asked her how she was doing with her new sport. "Oh, I stopped going," she said. "It was taking up too much of my time."

Well, I wasn't about to buy that, because one thing I've found to be true about Nancy in all the years she's been my patient: if she really wants to do something, she'll find the time—and whatever else she needs—to do it. Besides, she was obviously upset about it, and I wanted to find out why.

It turned out that the club she had joined was her first experience with a locker room. She had never been in a room with dozens of women running around naked before. For the first time in her life, Nancy was aware that all women don't have elongated labia. She was embarrassed about her body. The sad thing is that she was so busy worrying about the fact that she was different from everybody else that she didn't notice that all the women in the room were also different from everybody else. She was sure her labia were abnormal. It took a lot of convincing on my part to get her to see that there is simply no such thing as "normal" labia.

Worrying about the labia seems to be the female counterpart of the male worrying about the size of his penis. If that's been on your mind, relax. There is no such thing as labia that are the "wrong" size. What you have is right for you. (The same goes for the penis, by the way. We'll talk about that later on in this chapter.)

Starting at the top, the labia minora come together and form a covering or hood for the clitoris. The clitoris varies in size, and I'd like to stress that there is no "normal" size. It can be anything from a tiny nubbin that can't be seen because it's covered by the hood to a very large projecting clitoris that looks almost like a small penis. The clitoris is the seat of 90 percent of the sexual sensitivity in the female. The clitoris usually extends outside the hood, but occasionally the hood completely covers it. In those very rare instances when the hood can't be retracted, there can be a problem of decreased sensation. If that's the case, a circumcision can be done on the hood just as is done on the foreskin of the penis.

You don't see that done very often now, though it used to be fairly common. Before the pioneering research of Masters and Johnson, it was thought that the penis had to make direct contact with the clitoris in order to stimulate it. But Masters and Johnson found that as the penis moves in and out of the vagina, it moves the hood with it—and the hood stimulates the clitoris.

Just below the clitoris is a small opening called the urethral meatus, through which the woman urinates. The location of the meatus (the distance below the clitoris) varies from woman to woman. Below that is the opening of the vagina, which is usually ringed by irregularly shaped tissue—the remnants of the hymen, or maidenhead. The vagina also varies in distance from the clitoris. The lining of the vagina has many corrugations, or folds, and is usually moist.

I'm sure everybody knows that no two women have the same size or shape breasts. However, did you know that the great majority of women have one breast that's bigger than the other? If you've noticed that on yourself and you've worried that you're not normal, you can just stop worrying right now. Trying to find a "normal" pair of breasts would be like trying to find a "normal" set of fingerprints—it can't be done.

As long as I'm talking about breasts, I'd like to point out that breasts are a secondary sexual characteristic, and they have nothing at all to do with your sexuality. So size makes absolutely no difference.

What happens to all those structures as a woman gets older?

In the older woman, the pubic hair becomes more sparse and turns gray. Interestingly enough, the pubic hair is usually the last of the body hair to turn gray. I heard a story once about an older woman who was in the shower room of a swimming pool. A younger woman who was also showering stared with amazement at the older woman's head of pure white hair and pubic hair as dark as her own. Finally the young one couldn't hold back her curiosity any longer. "I don't understand how your pubic hair can be so much darker than the hair on your head," she blurted. The older woman thought about it for a moment and pointed to her head. "I guess it's because this is what I worry with"—then pointing to her vagina— "and this is what I have fun with."

The labia majora in the older woman are not as full, because fatty tissue is usually lost throughout the body with aging. The labia minora thin out as well, for the same reason. The clitoris remains much the same, though it may shrink slightly in size. *But very little,* if any, sensitivity is lost in the clitoris because of age.

The urethra might "pout" a little from the relaxation of the supporting muscles. Some women may have a small red growth on the rim of the urethra called a caruncle. A caruncle looks like a tiny wart or pimple, and it may be a cause of painful intercourse and a burning sensation when urinating. However, it is a condition that is easily cured. In fact, it can usually be taken care of right in the doctor's office. What we do is cauterize it. Cauterizing is burning, and it can either be done chemically with something like silver nitrate, or it can be done with an electric needle. After that's done, the patient is given a medicine to make the urine non-irritating. The whole thing heals in a week to ten days, and there is little or no discomfort during the healing period.

The vagina also changes with aging. The vaginal opening shrivels and narrows down. The lining of the vagina loses its folds, and the natural moisture decreases or disappears completely.

It's interesting to note that there are ways to keep those aging changes from happening—and regular sexual activity is one of them.

Now let's look at the male sex organs. Again, I'll talk about the younger male first, and then tell you what changes take place with age. This time, we'll start at the bottom.

First of all is the scrotum, a fairly firm sac in which you can feel a testicle on each side. You'll want to be careful if you do try to feel it, because the testicles are very tender. That's something I know any man is going to be familiar with, because it's impossible to get through life without being hit there at least once. You know, getting hit in the testicles is really an unpleasant thing, and the pain is so severe that it's easy to believe some real damage was done. I know most men believe a direct blow or a forceful squeeze can ruin or at least break a testicle. Well, it is possible, but a blow direct enough to do that is so rare you don't really have to worry. If you get hit there, it's going to hurt like the very devil, but it's not likely to do any lasting damage. Athletes get hit there frequently, and it doesn't turn them into eunuchs.

Another thing about the testicles—they are frequently not equal in size (either one can be the larger), and that's why one of them hangs lower than the other. If you were afraid you were abnormal because of that, don't be.

Now to the penis. The shaft of the penis seems to emerge from the top of the scrotum, and the shaft varies in length and diameter from one man to another.

This may be a good time to stop and talk about one of the biggest fears men have about sex. You know the one I mean—the one that goes, "Is my penis big enough?" Unfortunately, that's something all too many men worry about. No matter how often they are told otherwise, a lot of men still believe the size of the penis has a great deal to do with how well they perform sexually.

Masters and Johnson and many other sex researchers have proven conclusively that you can't tell by looking at a flaccid penis how long it's going to be when it is erect. They have also shown that the amount of erection is actually greater with a small penis. So what happens is the final difference in length usually varies from a half inch to an inch. The real difference in size is in the diameter. There are many men who have worried themselves into impotence because they have thin penises. The fact is, the diameter doesn't make a damn bit of difference, either. I think I've mentioned before that the female vagina can adapt to accommodate any size penis. That works both ways, you know. I didn't just mean it can stretch to accommodate a thick penis. I meant it can contract to accommodate a thin one as well. A female vagina is an amazingly elastic organ.

The myth still persists, though. I was talking about the problem with one of the guys I play golf with—another doctor, by the way—and he smiled kind of sheepishly and said, "I really believe size doesn't make a bit of difference, and I tell my own patients that all the time. But, Joe, every time I'm in the shower room at the club, I find myself surreptitiously checking out the plumbing on the other guys—and feeling jealous!"

There's an old saying that would be well for you to keep in mind: "It's not what you've got—it's how you use it." Another thing. No matter what you read in the men's magazines or hear from your friends, most women do not like exceptionally large penises. Why? Because they make intercourse uncomfortable, and sometimes even painful. Relax and be happy with what you've got. Your woman probably will be.

If a man has been circumcised, just where the skin ends is a little groove called the sulcus which forms the base of the head of the penis. The head of the penis is called the glans. Like the clitoris, this is a highly sensitive area. The opening of the urethra (called the meatus), through which you urinate, is at the tip of the head of the penis, and this opening can vary in size and sometimes position. Inside the shaft are three cylinders. The cylinders are honeycombed with tubes that fill with blood when the male is sexually excited. This filling with blood stiffens the penis and makes it erect. An easy way to see how that works is to take one of those long, thin balloons and watch what happens when you fill it with water.

The external organs don't really change much in an older man. The pubic hair becomes sparser and gray, the scrotum is looser, longer, and more wrinkled. The penis doesn't have the same firmness and hangs a little limper. The sensitivity of the head decreases slightly, but most of the sensitivity remains.

There are important organs in both sexes that are not visible. In the male there is the vas deferens, which is the pathway for the sperm from the testicles. The vas deferens runs through the prostate gland, alongside of which are two compartments called the seminal vesicles, where the sperm and the seminal fluid are stored prior to ejaculation. At the time of ejaculation, the vesicles and the ejaculatory ducts contract and squeeze the sperm and seminal fluid out through the urethra.

In the female, there is the uterus, which is in two parts, the body and the neck. The body of the uterus is in the pelvis, and the neck protrudes into the back end of the vagina. It's possible to feel the neck with a finger. Alongside the body of the uterus are the ovaries, where the ova (eggs) are produced. There is one ovary on each side. The ovaries are connected to the uterus by the Fallopian tubes. Those tubes are also known as oviducts, because they are the pathway for the ova to the uterus, where they are either fertilized by the sperm or discarded by the body in menstruation. Of course, once menopause has occurred, there is no more production of ova by the body, so the ovaries and the Fallopian tubes are no longer functional.

Those are the sexual tools you have. In the next chapter, I'll tell you how they work.

Chapter 3:
HOW YOUR SEX ORGANS WORK

Now that you know something about what your sex organs are, you may be wondering, "What can I do with them?" Or perhaps even, "Can I do *anything* with them?"

You most certainly can!

This point is so important, I can't stress it enough: given reasonably good health and a willing and stimulating partner, there is no good reason why sexual activity cannot be continued for a lifetime. That's right, a *lifetime!* I've already told you what I consider reasonably good health, and if you meet those standards, you're probably healthy enough to have sex.

You know you've got all the "tools" you need for sex, and you should have a pretty good idea of what they are and what they look like—especially if you've followed my advice and examined yourself (and your partner) carefully. If you haven't already done that, then use the previous chapter as a guide and do it now!

Ready? Then let's see how your sex organs work. This time, I'll discuss the man and the woman together. After all, sex is something you'll be doing together. As I did in the previous chapter, I'll begin my description with what happens to the younger person, and then show the changes that come with age.

It's been my experience that when people talk about the changes that come with age, they're trying to deal with some pretty formidable myths. They're trying to deal with concepts like, "You're over the hill." "What do you expect at your age?" "Those things are not for you anymore." In short, most people seem to believe that there is really only one big change when you get older—your sex organs just don't work anymore.

Let me assure you again that it's simply not true. There are changes in your body and the way you function sexually as you get older, but I think you'll be pleasantly surprised at how minor some of those changes are.

Masters and Johnson have divided the human sex cycle into four separate phases: 1) excitement, 2) plateau, 3) orgasm, and 4) resolution. In medical terms, the changes are produced by vasocongestion, myotonia, and decongestion. In simple terms, vasocongestion means the blood vessels of the genital area and other areas fill with blood. Myotonia means the muscles of the body tense, firm or tighten up, and decongestion means the blood vessels empty. Now let's go through each phase, one at a time, and see how that happens.

The Excitement Phase

That means exactly what it says—the body starts to get excited about the idea of having sex. In the earliest stages, the excitement can be triggered by the subtlest of stimuli, and any or all of the five senses can be involved. Have you ever been walking down the street and seen a good-looking woman or a handsome man and felt your pulse quicken? Well, that's one of the ways it can start. Or maybe the quickening comes from having your partner touch you or kiss you. Or maybe a random erotic thought pops into your mind, and you get an idea that it might be nice to cuddle with your partner and see what happens.

All those things make the body want to do something about it, and then the physical changes begin that make doing something about it possible.

The first thing that happens to a man is that the penis becomes erect. Remember those cylinders inside the penis we talked about before? Well, this is the time they fill with blood (vasocongestion), which makes the penis stiffen and get hard. That's likely to happen fast and with very little stimulus in a young man, especially if he is at an age near his sexual peak. I'm sure all of you men have at one time or another had the experience of getting an erection at an inappropriate and embarrassing time.

But there's a lot more to the excitement phase than an erection. A man might get goose pimples and the start of a skin flush. The skin flush is another result of vasocongestion. As the excitement phase continues, the skin covering the scrotum begins to get thick, and the testicles begin to rise in the scrotum. It's not unusual for a man to have some erection of the nipples. Toward the end of this first phase, breathing and the pulse rate get a little more rapid, and the tension begins to build up in the muscles of the body. That early tension is the start of myotonia.

Now what about you women? The first thing that happens when you get excited is the walls of your vagina begin to lubricate. In a younger woman, the lubrication can start as fast as the erection can start in a younger man. That's about ten to thirty seconds after stimulation begins. Along with the lubrication, the vaginal walls soften so the vagina can stretch to admit the penis when it is inserted. Later on in the excitement phase, the uterus raises, pulling on the vagina and making it longer.

A flush that looks like a rash starts under the rib cage and spreads quickly over the breasts. The nipples and the clitoris become erect. Blood flows to the various sex organs and turns the vaginal walls and the labia a deeper color. The change in color is caused by vasocongestion. As in the man, the woman's breathing and pulse quicken, and muscular tension builds up in the body (myotonia).

It's always been fascinating to me to see how well the body is made to work. For example, did you notice that the immediate reaction of both a man and a woman to sexual stimulus is the physical change most necessary to complete intercourse? In a man the first reaction is the erection of the penis so it can be inserted into the vagina; for the woman it is the lubricating of the vagina so it can accept the penis. All the other changes contribute something to the sexual act, but the first one is the one that counts the most.

That's also a good example of why it's important to "listen" to your body. Your body always knows what it wants, and it usually "tells" you in no uncertain terms. You may know that a formal dinner party is not the time or the place to get sexually excited—but if your body gets the right kind of sexual stimulus, it's going to react!

The Plateau Phase

If you say that the excitement phase is where the interest is shown, then the plateau phase is where the action takes place—most of the action, anyway. The excitement phase gets you *ready* to do something sexually, but this is where you actually *do* it.

The testicles continue to rise and move up closer to the body, and the scrotum gets even thicker and tightens. The penis is at its hardest and begins to throb. Breathing is heavier and faster, and the pulse is also much faster. Of course, by this time the penis has been inserted into the vagina.

The meatus (the opening in the urethra in the head of the penis) becomes wet from fluid from the prostate gland and vesicles. This fluid, or secretion, not only lubricates the urethral canal, but changes the environment to one which is favorable to sperm. You see, the urine flows out of the same place the sperm does. Urine is acid, and sperm can't live in an acid environment. So the fluid that lubricates the canal also changes the environment to an alkaline one, where the sperm can thrive. The change also makes the previously inactive and immobile sperm highly active and mobile. By this time, the thrusting, in-and-out movement of the penis has become more rapid.

Now the higher level of tension from all the added excitement shows up in the muscles. Men are likely to have involuntary spasms in the arms and legs (depending on what position you are in) and there will be twitches in the muscles of the face, neck, and abdomen as well. The thigh and buttock muscles of the male also contract during the last part of the plateau phase, which is a sign that orgasm is near.

During the plateau phase for women, the outer third of the vagina gets so swollen from blood that the vaginal opening actually becomes about a third smaller in size. The labia minora make their most dramatic color change, and the flush reaches its peak and spreads to all areas of the breasts, chest and abdomen, and sometimes to other parts of the body as well. This is the peak of vasocongestion.

In this phase, the clitoris pulls back completely into its hood. As it retracts, it goes out of reach of any kind of direct stimulation by finger or hand movements or by the thrusting penis. By the way, I included finger and hand stimulation because a woman can be brought to this phase (and, in fact, through all four phases) by manual manipulation. It doesn't have to be by intercourse. Why is it so important to remember that the clitoris retracts at this point? Because not knowing about it has caused a lot of frustration to a lot of people. Too many men have been told to keep stimulating the clitoris manually during foreplay and to keep the penis in contact with it during intercourse. I even gave you the example of a patient of mine earlier in the book who believed that myth. A man who tries to do it is begging to be frustrated, and get his partner frustrated as well.

But as Masters and Johnson have discovered, all that effort is completely unnecessary. The clitoris is stimulated without any special effort during intercourse. The thrust of the penis makes contact with the hood, which in turn puts pressure on the clitoris itself.

The Orgasm Phase

At this point, all the excitement that has been building up in the plateau phase comes to a peak. Breathing and pulse rates become even faster, more sweat appears, and the blood pressure rises.

In the male, the thrusting of the penis is at its most rapid, and then—ejaculation. The younger man has his ejaculation in two parts. Just before the actual emission of semen, he reaches a "point of no return." That's when he knows absolutely nothing in the world can keep him from ejaculating. Until that point he might be able to stop or be distracted, but once he reaches that point, its "Katie, bar the door!"

The second part of ejaculation is the emission itself. The thrusting of the penis becomes deeper and maybe slower, and often stops completely with one last, deep plunge at the moment of emission.

No one is quite sure yet exactly what triggers orgasm in a woman, so you women still have a little bit of an air of mystery about you. Orgasm for the woman can be defined as the release of muscle tension and swelling in blood vessels which builds up during the first two phases. But that sounds kind of dry and technical, doesn't it? A better way to think of orgasm is that it's the peak or ultimate in physical and emotional pleasure, with emphasis on the latter.

The female orgasm begins with rhythmic contractions (myotonia) in the outer third of the vagina that decrease in intensity and frequency after the first few. Uterine contractions may occur, which resemble menstrual cramps and can be painful. All female organs are not the same, so don't worry about meeting some mythical "standard." There is no standard orgasm. And the orgasm you have doesn't need to be a bell-ringer every time. Some women also have a spasm in the vagina that lasts as long as four seconds before the contractions start, almost like the "point of no return" feeling in a man just before he ejaculates.

The Resolution Phase

The body has reached its peak, and now it begins to come down. There is a general return to normal in the pulse and in the breathing, and the muscles of the body gradually relax. Organs swollen with blood return to normal (decongestion), and the penis and the clitoris lose their erections.

So those are the four parts of the human sex cycle. The whole process is something like putting on a teakettle:

First you turn on the stove and the water starts to get hot. That's excitement.

Then the water starts to boil and the steam builds up. That's the plateau.

And when the steam builds up enough so the kettle lets out a whistle—that's orgasm!

Finally, you turn the fire off, the steam dies down, and the water gradually cools. And that is resolution.

Now suppose you put salt in the water—what would happen? Exactly the same thing that would happen without the salt, but it would take a little longer. Think of your age as the salt in the boiling water, while I repeat something I said in the first chapter: everything that happens when you are young happens when you get older. It just happens slower. That's the only important difference between your sexual cycle and that of a younger person. But you still go through those same four stages.

The excitement state is prolonged for you older men, because it takes you longer to get an erection. Frankly, that's not such a bad thing. At least it keeps you from getting one at the wrong time. When you do get an erection, it won't be as rigid, but that doesn't matter. The woman can adapt to it easily. You may not get the skin flush or the rising of your testicles, and you won't get to the plateau phase as quickly, either. Things slow down and take longer at the plateau phase, too. Your movements won't be as vigorous as those of a younger man, but believe me, they'll be more than adequate.

When it comes to your orgasm, the big difference you'll notice is that there's only one stage. You won't have that feeling of being at a point of no return. You just keep going until you're there. It is going to take you longer to reach ejaculation.

The last phase—resolution—is the one exception to the general slowdown. There is no gradual relaxing of muscle tension and loss of erection; those things happen almost immediately. It also may take you several hours or even days to get another erection.

I hope all the talk about everything slowing down doesn't

make you feel disappointed about your prospects, because you shouldn't be disappointed at all. In fact, as I always tell my patients, there is an advantage you may not have thought of: the slowing down is going to make you a better lover. The longer period of foreplay can mean a much more stimulated and responsive partner. And without the urgent need to ejaculate that a younger man feels, you'll be able to stay with it long enough to be sure of satisfying your woman.

Here's something you may not be aware of: it's not necessary for you to ejaculate every time you have intercourse. I'll explain that and go into more detail about it in a later chapter, but for now I'll just ask you to take my word for it. The thing is, even without orgasm, you can still have a lot of fun. If you only ejaculate when you really need to, you are going to be able to have intercourse more often, because it won't take you as long to get erect again. This is the major difference between younger and older men.

Things are slowed down for the older woman, too, so you don't have to worry about one of you getting ahead of the other.

A younger woman will begin to lubricate within ten to thirty seconds of stimulation, but you older women might need from one to three minutes of non-demanding stimulation to achieve enough lubrication. It also takes longer for the clitoris and the nipples to get erect, and there may not be a sexual flush at all. In the plateau phase, your vagina won't expand as much, and it won't be as elastic, particularly if there has been a long period of abstinence.

There are a couple of things I'd like to talk about at this point: loss of elasticity and the drying out of the vagina. These are two of the negative effects aging has on the sexual organs of the woman. There are a couple of reasons why those problems happen. One is the decrease in the female hormone, estrogen, after menopause. The other cause is a lack of regular sexual stimulation. This is a good example of what "use it or you'll lose it" really means.

There are also a couple of ways to correct those conditions. The easiest one is to keep up sexual stimulation. I'm not sure exactly how it works, but I do know that it stimulates hormones to replace the ones you lost as a result of menopause. The other way to treat those problems of aging is to use artificial hormones—to administer estrogen, either orally or locally in the form of a cream. Estrogen has turned out to be a controversial subject, so maybe I should take the time right now to explain some things about it.

You've probably seen articles about estrogen in the magazines and newspapers you read. The subject has been discussed at great length in professional medical publications as well. I'm afraid the main thing that has come out of all the discussion is confusion. Some authorities praise estrogen to the skies, while others damn it as being downright dangerous.

As you may know, the problem is the possible link between estrogen and cancer. While we have no definite proof that estrogen can produce cancer where cancer does not exist, we do know that estrogen can stimulate the growth of a latent, resting cancer, either in the breast or in the uterus.

There are two ways of administering estrogen, you know, and each method gives different results. One way is to apply an estrogen cream to the affected area—the vagina. There is very little risk with local estrogens, and they do the job quite well. That is, they will effectively cure the dryness in the vagina. The solution to the controversy would seem to be a simple one then, wouldn't it? Unfortunately, no. Locally applied estrogen has one major drawback—it only works on the specific place it is applied. Which means that locally applied estrogen might help repair the dryness in the vagina, but it would do nothing for any of the other symptoms of menopause and aging.

Now I use oral estrogens in my own practice. I know there is a certain amount of risk involved, but when I prescribe the hormone treatments, I do it because I believe the benefits far outweigh the negative aspects. I'm also very, very careful about evaluating the patient I'm considering giving them to. There are certain guidelines that have been established for the use of estrogen in post-menopausal women.

First of all, there must be no history of cancer of the breast or uterus in her family among her female relatives as far back as her grandmother. That includes her mother, aunts, or any sisters. Cousins are not a factor in this kind of evaluation.

Women who have had a hysterectomy and no history of breast cancer are at little or no risk. And there must also be no history of blood clotting in the legs—or anywhere else in the body, for that matter.

Clots can develop after an operation, and they can develop after delivery of a baby. In those cases, I would absolutely not give oral estrogen at all.

After the family history, there's another factor I consider carefully before I make my decision. I have to be sure the patient is one who will cooperate by coming in for regular examinations and periodic pap smears. Why is that important? I mentioned before that we know oral estrogen can stimulate a cancer that already exists. Well, there is no way to tell if a woman has a latent cancer. The only thing a doctor can do is keep an eye on her, which is why I won't give it if I don't think the patient is a responsible person.

No matter how careful I am, though, the whole thing is still a calculated risk. If I have any doubts at all, I don't use the oral estrogen. And when I do use it, I use the smallest possible dose that will get rid of the symptoms. I also try to duplicate the natural cycle, that is, three weeks on estrogen and one week off.

If I feel a patient can use estrogen, I discuss it with her carefully. I explain the controversy about it, I point out the dangers, and I answer any questions she might have.

That's the best advice I can give you, because it is such an individual thing, you see. It's something that has to be decided between you and your doctor. Discuss the matter with him, ask all the questions you want to ask, and be sure you get answers that satisfy you.

If, after you have talked to your doctor, you are still not satisfied, don't hesitate to seek a second opinion.

I think that's enough about estrogens now. Let's go back to where we were before I digressed and talk about the effects of aging on the sexual cycle.

When you get older, your orgasms are going to be shorter. All that means is they won't last as long—it certainly doesn't mean they won't be satisfying. Believe me, they will be! Women can be multi-orgasmic at any age, which is a distinct advantage for those who wish to experience simultaneous orgasm. The first orgasm can be brought about by manual, oral, or mechanical stimulation, and the following ones by intercourse itself. Or, because older men tend to take much longer to reach orgasm and may lose and regain an erection several times, the order can be reversed.

The other big difference in your orgasm is that the vaginal contractions might not be as vigorous, or they might not occur at all. You might also not suffer the painful uterine contractions of the younger woman.

The resolution stage for the older woman is pretty much the same as that of the older male, except in multi-orgasmic women.

So that's how your sex organs work. And they do work and work well—as you can find out for yourself.

I can hear some of you men out there saying, "But mine doesn't work. What can I do about it?" Well, that's just what I'm going to start talking about next.

Chapter 4:
WHY YOU MEN MIGHT THINK YOU'RE IMPOTENT

If there is one word in the English language that is sure to fill a man with dread, that word is "impotence." Just the thought of it is enough to make you shrivel up, isn't it? Well, you're not alone. I seriously doubt if there's a man alive who hasn't at least experienced the *fear* of impotence, if not the actual failure to perform. Indeed, the word itself, with all that's associated with it, is in some disrepute, and some professionals prefer not to use it, and call it simply "male sexual dysfunction."

What exactly is impotence? That depends on whom you ask. I know of at least fifty definitions, and there are probably some I've never heard of, although my own patients have come up with some real lulus from time to time.

A man may think he's impotent because he can't have an orgasm more than once a night. A man may think he's impotent because he can't maintain an erection for twenty minutes. Another may think he's impotent because he isn't always in the mood when his wife wants him to be. I heard one man complain of impotence because his sexual drive is lower than that of his friends. They brag that they can go three or four times a night. Well, he can't, so he feels he's not normal.

And if he's not normal, he must be impotent. Yet another patient of mine is absolutely convinced he's impotent because he gets a much greater thrill from masturbating than he does from intercourse. If he has a problem, it certainly isn't impotence.

What does all that prove? Simply that everybody has his own ideas about what impotence is. Much of it seems to boil down to a vague concept called "being normal." When it comes to sex, most men are really afraid to be thought different. As a result, they tie themselves up in knots worrying about things that have nothing whatever to do with being normal, and nothing whatever to do with impotence, either.

At this point, it might be a good idea to leave the realm of myth and fantasy and find a good scientific definition of impotence. To my mind you can't find a better source for that definition than Masters and Johnson.

To begin with, Masters and Johnson have defined two basic kinds of impotence—primary and secondary. Primary impotence means a man has *never* been able to have an erection sufficient to perform a sexual act. Secondary impotence means a man *has* functioned sexually, and then fails. When I say he fails, I don't mean just once or twice, but at least fifty percent of the time.

Now here's something that might be a surprise to you. Only between 5 and 10 percent of what is called secondary impotence is due to physical or medical causes—what we call organic causes.

What do I mean by organic causes? I mean traumatic causes, such as direct injury to the genital area by an accident or severing of nerves in the genital area during surgery (in a radical prostectomy, for example). Other organic causes are congenital birth defects, absence of male hormones, or a badly deformed penis. Then there are the diseases which strike at the nerves, such as a tumor of the spinal cord or brain, traumatic severing of the spinal cord by accident, multiple sclerosis, strokes, and many cases of diabetes, which interrupt the flow of nervous energy to the sexual organs. Chronic alcoholism and many drugs (such as tranquilizers and drugs for treating high blood pressure) can also cause problems.

While these conditions can produce total impotence in some

cases, most of the time that doesn't happen, and the impotence that does occur can be treated successfully. I'll be telling you more about that later, when we talk about treating sexual disorders, but let me give you an example of what can be done about a case of impotence caused by surgery. One of the three sources of nerve supply to the sex organs is in the sacral area. The nerve endings are located in the capsule of the prostate. When a radical prostectomy is done, the capsule has to be removed, and those nerves are cut. However, in about 25 percent of the patients who have that operation, the other two nerve centers literally take up the slack and make sexual functioning possible again.

What happens in those and other cases is the man becomes partially impotent. It is possible to be partially impotent, because you can't destroy the libido, or desire for sex, just by destroying the nerve supply. The result might be that you can't get an erection, but you can still ejaculate. You don't need an erection to ejaculate.

If only 5 to 10 percent of impotence is organic, that still leaves 95 percent or so to be accounted for. If that 95 percent isn't in your body, where do you suppose it is? Right! It's in your head. That's why I don't really like to use the word "impotence," because 95 percent of the time the problem isn't impotence at all—it's simply failure to perform. I've said this to you before, but it bears repeating: the most important sex organ lies between the ears, not between the legs.

Failure is from the collar up, not from the waist down. If you can't perform, chances are your mind and not your body is causing it. So the first time you have trouble getting an erection, if you say, "What's wrong?" you've taken a big step toward failure.

Now, contrary to what you might have heard or what you might think, that kind of failure doesn't begin when you're a senior citizen. It usually happens in middle age, because that's the time of your life you are most likely to be faced with a heavy load of stress. A common source of that stress is pressure from your job or your business. One of my patients, a man barely into his forties, is a good example of that.

Harry was the owner of a manufacturing company in a

highly competitive field that employed 1,500 people. He came into my office and blurted out that he was impotent, and he wanted to know why. He thought he was far too young for such a thing to happen, and I agreed. "In fact," I told him, "Harry, I think your dad is far too young for that kind of thing to happen." He wasn't too sure how he felt about *that*, but he knew he wanted to take care of his own problem. I asked him, "What time do you get to work?" and he said, "About seven o'clock, but I usually can manage to get a lot done while I'm having my coffee at home, and I keep a tape recorder in the car for dictating letters and memos so I don't waste the hour it takes for me to drive to the plant."

Harry not only started working almost the minute he got up in the morning, but he more often than not ate his lunch at his desk while he got even more accomplished. On top of everything else, he never left the office until seven or eight at night. "I suppose you take work home with you, too," I said. "Of course, I do," he replied. His employees, on the other hand, worked a normal day, took a coffee break in the morning and another in the afternoon, and had a regular lunch hour.

I told him, "You expend a tremendous amount of mental and emotional energy during your working day, which is every bit as exhausting as physical energy. Then the evening comes and you think it might be a good idea to have sex with your wife. Not because you really want to have sex, but you want to show her that you are still interested in her and you still care for her. You make a try, but your mind is really still on your business, so you fail. The fact that you are doing it more or less as a duty instead of something you really want to do for its own sake is more than likely to result in failure."

Then I asked him, "What happens when you go on vacation?"

"Oh, I'm not too bad on vacation," he said. "In fact, I do pretty well."

"Doesn't that tell you something?" I asked. I then told him that he was going to have to cut down drastically on the amount of work he did and take some of the pressure off himself or he would really have a problem when he got older. That kind of problem starts in middle age, and by the time a man has gotten older, he's beginning to use it as an excuse for not functioning sexually.

Here's another way that first failure could happen. Suppose you have had a long night of drinking. Alcohol is a notorious sexual depressant, and you just can't get it up. You really want to do it, and your partner really wants you to do it, but you fail.

The sensible thing to do would be to try it again in the morning when you are sober. But suppose you don't do that. Suppose you are a little scared, so you wait until later in the day, and then you have a few drinks to get up your courage. Once again the alcohol depresses your ability to perform, and you fail for the second time.

That second failure intensifies your fear of failure, and from then on you're really going to be anxious. Anxiety and fear are the basic causes of impotence. The more you give in to anxiety and fear, the more failures you will have, and it won't be long before you look down at your limp penis and ask, "Why did you have to die before me?" Now here's an amazing thing: many men who are absolutely convinced they are impotent have absolute proof they can still function sexually. They just don't recognize the proof for what it is. What's the proof? *They wake up in the morning with an erection!*

"All right," you might say, "I wake up with an erection. But if I try to use it, the damn thing dies. And if I want to have intercourse later, I can't even get an erection."

There are a lot of reasons for that, which have nothing at all to do with impotence. The reason might be simply that your wife isn't interested then, and her attitude makes you lose the erection. That kind of thing happens to younger men, too, you know. Or maybe she is willing to try, but her responses have slowed down and she can't wake up out of a sound sleep and get her vagina lubricated and ready for you in the blink of an eye. So there's a lot of fumbling around and frustration, and your body loses interest. Or maybe you lose the erection because you're trying too hard and you scare it away.

What I'm trying to tell you is that your body is not playing a cruel joke on you with that morning erection—it's telling you the truth about yourself. There's an old saying that has been proven time and again, "The body never lies." What your body is telling you is that when you're relaxed and not worrying about it, you really are capable of functioning sexually. But if you ignore the obvious evidence of your body telling you it's possible, then you're playing a cruel joke on yourself. As Masters and Johnson have said, "What nature deals out to man is kindness compared to what man deals out to himself."

However, the question that's probably burning in your mind right now is—can I be cured?

You most certainly can! That's one of the major goals of this book, to show you how to do it. Just bear in mind that if you are failing to perform sexually for psychological reasons, you can probably be helped. Before we can talk about how to cure your sexual problem, you have to understand something about what the problem is, and what could be causing it.

I don't have to tell you you're getting older. You know that. I'd be willing to bet almost anything that "getting older" is the biggest thing on your mind right now. That's why I don't like to ask my patients how old they are chronologically. Instead, I ask them, "If you didn't know your chronological age, how old do you think you would be?" The answer to that question usually gives me a pretty good clue to how successful the man is going to be in overcoming his problems.

I get some interesting reactions to that question, by the way. One guy I know who is making the most of his retirement told me, "I don't even think of my age. I play eighteen holes of golf a day, and then I come in and swim thirty or forty laps in the pool. My wife and I go dancing a couple of times a week, and I'm having a ball." Then I asked him about his sex life, and do you know what he said? "I don't do that anymore. You know, a guy my age, it's not right to be thinking about that stuff all the time like I was some young kid or something."

Funny, isn't it? I'm that man's doctor, so I know what kind of shape he's in and just how good his health is. Believe me, if he's not having sex, it's because he doesn't want to for some reason, not because he can't. Of course, he is impotent, but he's impotent by choice. The only thing needed to make him function is to get him to understand how ridiculous it is for him to act like "some young kid or something" everyplace but the bedroom. However, his success with his other activities at his age does prove my point—you're as young as you think you are.

It works the other way, too. You can also be as *old* as you think you are. I get plenty of men dragging themselves into my office to tell me something like, "Well, doctor, what can I expect at seventy? I'm going downhill, anyway. How much longer can I live? Another year, another two years. My time is limited; every day is a bonus. I'm not ready to die, but I've got to look it in the face."

That kind of person walks around with a doom-and-gloom attitude, as if he expects every day to be his last. He's doing everything he can to make himself miserable, and all that's going to do is make the end come faster. He might have five years, or ten years left, but he's not going to be happy. The older he gets, the more convinced he's going to be that the next day is going to be his last.

That attitude is more common in somebody who has been ill. His doctor might tell him he's all right, but he worries about getting sick again. He can't convince himself he's well. There's not very much chance for him to be able to function sexually. What has to happen with him is you have to convince him that as long as he doesn't know how much time he has left, he might as well enjoy every day of it. If that happens, maybe he'll think, "I might have five or six years to go, and there's a lot of fun to be had in five or six years!"

How about you? How old do *you* feel? And how much time do you spend thinking about all the things you're afraid you can't do anymore because you're "too old?" What happens when you see a good-looking woman walking down the street? Do you let yourself have a harmless, enjoyable fantasy about her—or do you just sigh and mutter, "Them days are gone forever!"

Maybe you feel you're no longer the stud you used to be. Your responses are slower, and you don't have the strength or agility you had when you were younger. So you think you're going downhill, and you start to feel old. Along with feeling old comes the belief you can no longer function sexually. The fact is, aging *does* bring a slowing down of all your bodily functions, including sex. I know I've said it before, but it does bear repeating: slowing down does not mean stopping. It doesn't even mean the beginning of the end. All it means is that some things take a little longer than they used to.

It's pretty easy to misunderstand the normal changes in your body and believe you're over the hill. Unfortunately, if that's what you want to believe, you can find a lot of support for it. Some comedians and cartoonists are having a field day ridiculing the sex life of the older male. And let's not forget songs like "Too Old to Cut the Mustard." No wonder so many men are using age as an excuse for stopping sex. That's what it is, you know—an excuse. It's not aging that brings sexual activity to an end, but the *fear* of aging that brings on the fear of failure, and all the attitudes that go along with those fears.

What kind of attitudes? Well, attitudes about yourself, for example. About the way you look. Your personal appearance is often the best clue to how you really feel about yourself, and in many cases it determines how others are going to feel about you. How about it? Are you as careful about the way you look as you were when you were younger? Or have you let yourself go? Have you gotten careless about the way you dress, or how often you shave or bathe? Are you eating too much and putting on weight?

That kind of carelessness is a good way to make yourself old before your time. If you start to feel old, you're going to start to act old. Then you'll start to fail sexually, because you'll be evaluating your sexuality in terms of increasing age.

Being careless about how you look can work against you another way, too. It can really turn off what might otherwise be an interested and willing partner. Let me give you an example of how personal appearance can affect a woman's judgment of a man.

A woman I know—she's in her late twenties—works in an office with two men in their sixties. Harry is overweight; his clothes never seem to fit right and they are usually badly wrinkled. He often needs a shave and smells a little bit overripe. "He's a real slob," is the way the young woman describes him.

"Harry is always coming on with me," she says. "I can't talk to him for two minutes without getting propositioned half a dozen ways. Coming from him, that really annoys me. I've tried everything I can think of, including outright rudeness, to get him off that subject. You know, he comes on pretty strong, but I don't think he could do anything about it if his life depended on it."

Tom, on the other hand, is two years older than Harry, but there's a bigger difference between them than two years of age. Tom takes care of himself. His clothes are neat and well-fitting, and he keeps himself trim with regular exercise. "I get a kick out of flirting with Tom," my young friend says, "but he always responds by telling me, 'Honey, I'd love to, except that I'm old enough to be your grandfather.' Maybe he is, but he still looks kind of good to me."

The interesting thing about her evaluation of those two men is that she never once mentioned age. She based her whole opinion on the way they looked.

Now, it sounds like Tom is not only perfectly able to function sexually, he *is* functioning. What might happen if he decided to take advantage of the young woman's offer sometime? He's not married, so there's really no reason why he couldn't. He might not try because he would be afraid of going against the so-called "norm" for men his age—he's afraid of being laughed at. He's afraid of being called a "dirty old man."

You know, that's a hell of a nasty expression, and it's one I don't like very much. But it sure is common. Anybody, from your children to your best friend, is likely to throw it at you. If you try to protest that you don't fit into that category, you're likely to be accused of bragging—or told people your age shouldn't be thinking such "nasty" thoughts.

All too often, younger people think sexual activity in the older population is negligible, unimportant, or non-existent. In fact, to hear some young people talk, you'd think they were all conceived through virgin birth.

Children usually go through four stages in their attitudes toward their parents having sex: when they are very young, they say, "There's no such thing!" As they get a little older, that changes to, "Well, maybe there is such a thing, but *they* don't do it!" When they reach maturity, they believe and accept the fact that their parents engage in sex. Then, as those children approach middle age (and their parents become senior citizens), it's right back to, *"They* don't do it!"

What effect does this attitude have? It conditions people to act as if it were true. As they come to believe it, they withdraw more and more from sexual contact until they reach the point where they do it rarely or they stop completely.

However, the desire to change those attitudes is very much in the air. I see that desire every time I lecture on this subject. The intense interest displayed by my audiences of older people and the delighted glances they give each other tell me plainer than anything else could how eager they are to rid themselves of those archaic, obsolete attitudes about their sexual behavior, mores, and desires.

What about you? Isn't it about time you stopped worrying about what other people might be thinking? Isn't it about time you stopped believing the whole world is watching every move you make, ready to point an accusing finger if you do something *they* think is wrong or unacceptable? If you think more of the attitudes of others than your own needs, you may very well find yourself unable to perform sexually.

It might be interesting and, in fact, comforting to know that with each succeeding lecture I find more and more young people in my audiences. They seem to be delighted at my insistence that sex can go on for years to come, that something which is an important part of their lives now will continue to be an important part of their lives in the future.

People in your age group are more likely to have had a fairly strict upbringing. Or maybe you called it an "old-fashioned" upbringing, which means the same thing. I'm not saying the old-fashioned way was all bad. But the fact is, some of the things you were taught in your youth can stand in the way of sexual fulfillment now—fulfillment you have every right to enjoy as long as you want to.

For example, were you taught that sex is for procreation and never for recreation? If you believe that, then you could easily believe that when you get to a certain age, you should be through with sex. Or do you feel guilty because you want to give in to what you were taught was an animal urge? Or do you feel guilty because you were taught that looking at a woman's naked body with a lustful eye was a sin?

One of the saddest stories I ever heard was of a woman in rural Georgia who had just buried her husband. The area where she lived didn't have an undertaker, so they still held to the old custom of the family preparing the body for burial. This woman, who had been married for almost sixty years, said she first discovered her husband had a birthmark when she washed his body for burial.

It makes me sad to think of the frustration and human waste those mid-Victorian attitudes still cause. No, it doesn't just make me sad—it makes me mad as hell to see potentially vital, happy people turn into bitter, decrepit shells.

Many older people who are perfectly willing to have sex are faced with the loss or lack of a partner. Maybe that's the case for you. What can you do? How can you satisfy your sexual needs and stay active enough sexually so you don't lose the capability you have? There is an easy, logical, and healthy solution to those problems, but guilt and shame might be keeping you from using it.

As you probably guessed, I'm talking about masturbation. Masturbation has been a lively moral issue for years, with parents and churches preaching its evils. Just a list of all the myths about how harmful masturbation is could fill another book. Maybe it's time somebody told you the truth about masturbation. It's harmless, it's normal, it's healthy, and it's a good way to keep from drying up if you can't have sex with a partner. In other words, it's a damn good way to use it, so you don't lose it!

Sex researchers have proved over and over again that virtually every male alive either has masturbated, is masturbating now, or is going to masturbate as soon as he's old enough. But if any of the stories you've always heard are true, the masturbators should be easy to spot. They'll be the ones with the hairy palms and warts all over their bodies. If you look around, you should be able to see dozens of them, at least. Not one? Amazing, isn't it?

There's another twist to the masturbation myths that's kind

of interesting. I'm talking about the warnings against "excessive" masturbation. You may have been told, "If you do that too much, you won't have it when you need it." I had a man in his early twenties come to me with that problem. He was having intercourse at least once a day, plus masturbating three or four times a week. He had begun masturbating when he was about eleven, and he was really worried that he was going to run out of something and not be able to have sex when he was older. He thought he was squandering his sexual future. I was quick to assure him that the result of all that activity now was almost sure to be a vigorous sex life when he got older.

The funny thing is, a lot of people do believe that excessive masturbation can be harmful—but you can't get any two of them to agree on how much is "excessive."

When Masters and Johnson threw the question at some of their test subjects, they got some surprising answers. The frequency of masturbation among the subjects ranged from once a month to several times a day. But no matter how often anyone did it, he defined "excessive" as *more* than he was doing. For the once-a-month masturbator, twice a month was excessive. For someone doing it four times a day, "excessive" was something like six or seven times a day.

Not one of the men questioned thought his own masturbating was excessive. Obviously the old saying, "Enough is too much," doesn't apply here!

Another relic from the dusty past that can cause sexual failure is the mistaken belief that the man has all the responsibility for sex. We've been taught for too long that the man is the one who is supposed to take the lead in sexual matters. He has to start it, take part in it, and finish it satisfactorily. That's a lot of responsibility to heap on one half of what should be a shared partnership. It puts a tremendous strain on a man. And all too many men begin to fail sexually when they try too hard to live up to that responsibility. The pressure to perform is even more intense nowadays, because more and more women believe they are entitled to sexual satisfaction and are demanding it from their sexual partners.

It isn't what you do as the man to or for the woman or what the woman does to or for you—it's what you do for each other for mutual pleasure and for which together you take full responsibility. If you succeed, you have created an ideal relationship; if you fail, it's neither your fault nor the fault of your partner. Somewhere you have simply failed to communicate your likes and dislikes, your fears, your inhibitions or restrictions to your freedom of action in your sexual relations.

Pressure from outside can cause sexual failure, too, as I pointed out earlier in this chapter. As I said in a slightly different context, just about the time you begin to worry about your sex life—in later middle age—is the time when you're most likely to be at the peak of success in your business life, with all the extra worries that can bring. The pressure of business, the pressure of maintaining a certain standard of living, take up most of your physical and emotional energy. It's fairly common for a man at that time to have some trouble functioning sexually, while his mind and body adjust to all those added drains on his energy.

That's the crucial point in a man's sex life. That's the time real sexual failure may or may not take hold.

If you realize that the pressure of business has taken up so much energy you can't relax enough for sex, and don't let it get to you, your problems will most likely go away in time. But if there is even a momentary thought that you are beginning to fail, then that's the first sign of real failure.

That happened to one of my patients when he was about sixty-three. He had been doing fine sexually, but one night he failed. Right away, he got worried, and instead of just forgetting about it, he had it on his mind all the next day. So the next night he was determined to perform, because he had failed the night before. Now his mind was on failure, not on how much fun he was going to have. It was serious business all of a sudden. He had to see if he was going to be any good.

As I've said before, it's impossible to will an erection, which was what he was trying to do. Needless to say, it didn't work. After the fifth or sixth failure, his wife became very aware that he was worried about it. Instead of discussing it calmly, however, she said, "I think you better get to a doctor." That was actually good advice, but the way she said it planted the seed of another doubt in his mind. She reinforced his fear that there was something wrong with him.

Unfortunately, the doctor he was seeing at the time was not well-versed in the problems of human sexuality. Besides that, he was well along in years himself. After a perfunctory examination, the doctor simply said he couldn't find anything physically wrong, "but you can't really expect to be like you used to be, at your age."

That was enough to drive the final nail. The man was made impotent by the cumulative effect of three separate incidents: first, his own notion that there was something wrong; second, his repeated attempts and failures, reinforced by his wife's belief there was something wrong; and third by the doctor telling him something was wrong and he was too old to get it fixed.

The man has since been referred to me for treatment, and among other things, I have gotten him into therapy.

I'd like you all to keep one thing in mind. You *will* fail from time to time. Everybody does. But remember—the ability to function sexually is there.

And there's always a next time.

Chapter 5:
FRIGIDITY AND WHY WOMEN FAIL TO RESPOND SEXUALLY

Now that we've dealt with impotence in men, it's time to talk about the equivalent problem you women may have to deal with. That's right—I mean frigidity. And again, this is an old-fashioned word for "sexual dysfunction."

What do I mean when I say "frigidity" or female sexual dysfunction? Well, the term is much like the term "impotence" for men, and there are about as many myths and definitions as there are for impotence.

Each woman has her own idea of what frigidity means. A woman might come in and say she's frigid because she doesn't get any feeling out of sexual experience, any excitement. She might admit to getting a great deal of satisfaction out of petting and stroking, but as long as there is no thrill from intercourse, she is frigid as far as she is concerned.

Many women believe they are frigid because they can only have orgasm by manual stimulation of the clitoris—it never happens to them from intercourse. I've even had a patient tell me she was frigid because she couldn't have her orgasm at the right time. "What do you mean, at the right time?" I asked her. "I mean I don't come at exactly the same time my husband does," she said. It turned out that she had no trouble having an orgasm every time she had intercourse. Her problem was she confused frigidity with simultaneous orgasm.

Other women think they are frigid because they are too tired to have intercourse every day, or maybe only like to do it in bed with the lights out.

So you can see from all this that frigidity means one thing to the woman, and another thing to the doctor. The term "frigidity," by the way, is gradually being replaced by most authorities on human sexuality with the term "sexual dysfunction." That's really a much more accurate way to describe the general problem. However, I think "frigidity" might be better for our purposes, because that's the word most of us are familiar with. An important thing to remember is that we're using a simple word to stand for a very complex problem. In other words, there is not just one kind of frigidity—there are several degrees of it.

Of course, it's been obvious for a long time and in many ways that men and women are different. One of the most interesting differences, to my mind, is the way they think of their sexual capabilities when they get older. Men want to have sex, but they aren't sure they are able. The women, on the other hand, know they are able, but they aren't sure they want to.

Yes, that is a little oversimplified, but it's not as far from the mark as you might think. With all the recent sex research and the popular articles that have come out of it, it has become common knowledge that you women reach your sexual peak much later in life than men do. Men reach that peak in their teens and early twenties, while women reach it in their late thirties and early forties.

In spite of that, a woman in our society is able to accept the idea of being frigid a lot more easily than a man can accept the idea of being impotent. A man's ego is very closely related to his sexual potency, but that's not entirely true for a woman. When a man feels impotence approaching or gets the first notion that he's having difficulty, it's a disaster to him. A woman can accept her loss of sexual excitement, her lack of sexual response, if she has become accustomed to a slowdown on the part of her husband. The idea of being content with less doesn't bother her as much as it bothers her husband. Of course, this is not always the case. And perhaps contemporary knowledge about sex and changing mores will change this, too, in time.

The most extreme kind of frigidity is what is called "primary sexual dysfunction," or "absolute sexual dysfunction." That describes a woman who has never in her lifetime been aroused in any way, shape, or form. In case you're not sure—when I say arousal, I mean the ability to be stimulated to the state of excitement that produces lubrication. Lubrication for a woman is the equivalent of an erection for a man. Just as it's occasionally possible for men to go through life without having an erection, so it is possible for a woman to go through her life without ever being aroused enough to become lubricated.

Granted, this is not a common problem. Generally, only an extremely rigid moral upbringing would cause that kind of problem. A woman with this problem would have to grow up with an aversion or even hatred of the very idea of sex. When she does come into contact with men as an adult, her attitudes are going to keep her from experiencing any kind of sexual arousal.

So much for the really extreme cases. There's another kind of primary sexual problem that's a lot more common—the woman who can be aroused enough to lubricate, but who never has had an orgasm. How does that happen? Mostly it comes from early training. For example, let's suppose that you were taught from childhood on that you were just meant to have babies, and you were not supposed to get any pleasure from sex. What's the result likely to be?

First of all, if you do start to feel any pleasure, you'll probably stifle it—and keep on stifling it until it becomes a behavior pattern. You'll eventually teach your body to have no sense of feeling at all. By the same token, if you did feel pleasure in sex but were always taught it was wrong to show it, you are likely to inhibit that pleasure until you get to the point where you become frigid.

As long as I'm telling you about the more serious problems,

I think I ought to tell you something about vaginismus. That means the muscles of the vagina contract so intensely that vaginal intercourse is not possible. A woman with vaginismus is usually able to be sexually aroused. She'll have all the feelings and emotions of arousal—she will lubricate, her nipples will become erect, her clitoris will erect, she'll have the flush. In short, she'll have all the signs. But the minute an attempt is made to enter the vagina, she subconsciously contracts every muscle of the vagina to the point where not even the tip of a finger can be inserted.

I'm treating a young woman with that kind of problem right now. Here's how it happened. She married a man in his late thirties, and it was the first marriage for both of them. She was a virgin when they were married, but as you might expect with the double standard, he was not. I would call her upbringing strict, but not unusually so. She had some fears about sex—almost every woman does at first, perhaps everyone does—but with an understanding and considerate partner, those fears were nothing that would have caused serious problems.

The first time a woman has intercourse is an important time for her, because she is very vulnerable emotionally. The first time can be much easier for a woman if the man has some experience. Unfortunately, it didn't work out that way with this couple. The man's only sexual experience was with prostitutes—not usually a good training ground for a loving sexual relationship.

Don't get me wrong—I think his intentions were all right. It was the way he carried them out that backfired. His idea of intercourse was, you get on, you hurry and do it, you get off. No preliminaries, and no cuddling afterward. And that's how he approached his bride for her first time.

Well, she was nowhere near ready for intercourse. She hadn't even started to lubricate when he tried to enter her, and he really hurt her badly.

She clamped up her vaginal muscles that first time, and she still clamps up every time he comes near her. They've been married for more than a year now, and he still has not been able to penetrate her. Technically, she's still a virgin. And to top the whole thing off, she's pregnant! Even though she has never been penetrated, the semen leaked through and she conceived.

You're probably wondering how that could happen. Sperm have a tendency to go uphill against the current. So it is very easy for sperm to enter the vagina, even though the ejaculation occurs on the outside, and then move up the cervical canal and meet an ovum which is ready to be fertilized. It's just like a salmon swimming upstream to spawn.

She has serious problems now, and it's going to take a lot of time and effort to overcome them. Would she be better off with a different man? Probably not. I don't think she could make herself trust another man any more than she does her husband right now, and trust plays a very important part in female sexual response.

Those problems are more likely to happen to younger women. They aren't really problems that pertain to aging as such. Why am I talking about them then? Because there are ways those problems could carry over into an older age, especially if you are an older woman who has never married. It could also happen to an older woman who has suffered a traumatic sexual experience in her adult life—a rape, for example, or an injury or surgery that caused her great pain.

There might be a woman who has had sexual intercourse and has been traumatized to the point where the thought of penetration causes real fear. Those problems can happen to anyone, and the older the problem is, the more difficult it will be to correct.

I've been saying a lot to you women about how much better sex is supposed to be for you as you get older. Many of you may be reading this and wondering why *you* simply don't care. A woman can mistake the failing sexual potency of her mate or the gradual development of impotence in him as a rejection, because she feels she is aging and that her appearance may be fading. She sees her partner going into a decline, and she blames herself for the decline. She says, "Look, I'm older and I'm not as attractive as I used to be, so he's rejecting me. He doesn't want me as much as he used to."

Frigidity and Why Women Fail To Respond Sexually 69

Of course, if you have the money, the time and the inclination, you can keep yourself looking young almost forever with cosmetic surgery and other specialized treatments. But that kind of thing really isn't necessary. There are plenty of ways you can keep yourself looking attractive without going to those extremes. If you take care of yourself, watch your weight, keep well groomed and dress attractively, you're going to look good. No, you're not going to look like a woman in her twenties, but that isn't what you need to do. All you need to do is look like an attractive person of your own age. Never discount the fact that you've been around for a while. For one thing, your life experience is going to give you a lot more to talk about. You are probably going to be a lot more interesting than any young woman after the first half-hour, and maybe earlier! And that's a good part of what attractiveness is—being interesting.

If you think the physical changes of age in you are causing your partner to have sexual problems it's really sad, because the decrease in the male sex drive is a natural thing that happens with age. You must understand that nature slows him down, and it has nothing to do with you. It's not your fault, and it's not a rejection. The changes are not the same for each sex.

If you've read the previous chapter, you'll be aware that your partner is going to slow down as he gets older. And if you haven't read the preceding chapter, do it now! You need to understand the problems your partner might have if you want to understand your own problems. I can't stress that point enough. The more you and your partner understand about each other, the more you are going to be able to express yourselves sexually.

As I said, the man's ability might diminish as he grows older, and that's a natural thing. However, it is not at all natural for a woman's desire to decrease with age. Most of the time any decrease in a woman's sexual appetite is due to a decrease in activity on the part of the man. That's what I meant when I said earlier in the book that it was usually the husband's responsibility when sex stopped.

Maybe your partner has slowed down and you have let

yourself slow down, too, in the mistaken belief that it's all part of the same aging process for both of you. I want to reassure you right now about that. No matter how slow your partner gets, *you* don't have to slow down at all. *You* don't have to feel any lessening of sexual response. That doesn't mean you won't have to make adjustments in your sex life, because you certainly will.

Let's not go into that right now, though, because I'll be talking about it in detail in a later chapter. But there are many ways, as you will see, for your partner to give you all the sexual satisfaction you need.

One of the things I've been saying in this chapter is that a decrease in sexuality because of age is not natural for a woman. I'd like to amend that statement, because there is a circumstance when it is natural. A woman may have been taught to believe that menopause means the end of her sexuality. If she really believes that to be true, then she is preconditioned to it, which does make it seem a natural thing for her, even though it's not a biological necessity.

The onset of menopause can be a critical time in your life. So let's suppose you have gone through menopause, and you have been told that your libido is supposed to be increasing. The trouble is, you just can't seem to get interested in sex anymore. One of the reasons could be that you were taught sex is for procreation, not for recreation. Oh, yes, that again! You have always thought of sex as a duty, and maybe even as a kind of prison you would be released from someday. If you've been counting the days until your release, of course you aren't going to be interested in continuing with sex. You've done your duty. You've served your time. You've been released from your "bondage." Now you can forget all about that stuff and relax.

That's something I see a lot of in my practice—a woman "does her duty" all her married life, and then when menopause comes, she feels relief that it's all over . . . and then maybe she is widowed. So what if such a woman meets another man after a while and romance blossoms? There is likely to be a sexual encounter to which she can't respond, and she doesn't understand why. This example isn't something I made up just

Frigidity and Why Women Fail To Respond Sexually

to prove my point. It really happens. It upsets me no end to think how *often* it happens.

I get angry at that, because by the time such a woman comes to me with the problem, it's already a serious one. The fact that she consults me at all shows she is interested in regaining her sexuality. But now, instead of a relatively simple correcting of misinformation and mistaken attitudes, it becomes a matter of retraining some pretty well-entrenched behavior patterns. That could be a long, drawn-out process. It's time she could have been spending in the enjoyment of sex. And all too often the woman will give up in frustration long before she can start to enjoy sex.

Those women who see the menopause as a release—and I've seen plenty of them in my years as a doctor—are classic examples of women who have never appreciated their sexual roles. The more severe and strict the upbringing, the worse the problem is going to be. Some backgrounds are virtual guarantees that a woman will grow up unable to appreciate her sexuality.

On the other hand, you may be very much aware of your increased desire for sex, or at least be starting to realize that increasing age doesn't have to mean decreasing sexual function. But if you have a partner whose dying ability to have sex often leaves you unsatisfied, you're going to find yourself gradually losing interest.

Which brings up something I've said several times before, and I promise you I'll be saying again—the most important element of a good sexual experience at *any* age is an interesting and *interested* partner. You'll notice I stressed the word "interested" just now.

A real *lack* of interest in the sense I mean was shown by the husband of a patient of mine. For years he was at her virtually every night—wham, bam, he was finished. She never did get a chance to find out that sex could be fun. Well, she put up with it as a duty until she went through menopause, and then—you guessed it—she dropped it like a hot potato!

That may not sound like lack of interest to you. The guy was after her almost every night, wasn't he? Sure he was, but he didn't really care about her satisfaction. She was just a tool for his sexual release, for the release of his tensions without regard for whether or not she got any release. Not that it was all his fault. She should have made it known long before that she was an individual and that she had her own needs. But her background and upbringing didn't allow her to do that, so she put up with sex as a duty.

As long as she was treating sex as a duty, there could be no pleasure in it at all for her. As soon as she could, she used an excuse (that he was uninformed enough to believe)—that once the menopause came, she was through sexually.

Of course, some of the reasons you might be feeling a lack of interest in sexual activity are going to be physical. Aging does change your body, and some things are simply not as comfortable for you to do as they once were. That's especially true if there has been a gap in your sexual activity. You've probably heard that a lack of sex will "dry you up," and maybe you've dismissed the idea as nonsense. Would you be surprised to know that it's true? That really is what happens to your body.

Stopping sexual activity can hasten the development of a condition called senile vaginitis, which is a drying and smoothing out of the tissues of the vagina. The vaginal wall gets thinner, there's difficulty lubricating. The lips of the vagina shrivel and flatten out. This condition lends itself to an increased risk of vaginal or bladder infections. Those physical changes are enough to drive any remaining sexual desire right out of most women.

Fortunately, something can be done about that condition. Part of the treatment is the use of estrogens, which I discussed earlier. The other part of the treatment is a lot easier, a lot less controversial, and frankly, a lot more fun—returning to sexual activity. The two of them together can completely reverse the aging of a woman's sex organs in a very short time.

It's a well-documented fact that continuing your sex life will keep you young sexually. But in spite of all the very good reasons for older women to be having the special joys of a fulfilling sexual relationship, all too many are not. I can almost

Frigidity and Why Women Fail To Respond Sexually 73

hear many of you saying, "How can I have a sexual relationship if I don't have somebody to have one with?" The lack of an available partner is a common problem. There may be any number of good reasons why you would find it difficult or even impossible to have regular sexual intercourse. In that case, the best solution is simply masturbation.

Let's stop for a moment so you can catch your breath. I know that word is a shock to a lot of you, and I know that some of you find the idea of masturbating unpleasant and even shameful. But it is a valid means of sexual activity, and when other ways are not available to you, it's a good way to keep yourself from drying up.

That's enough about masturbation for now. I think it's important enough to discuss at length, but that will wait for another chapter.

Keeping your sexuality is important, though. Maybe you find that a little hard to believe. I can hear some of you widows out there saying, "What for? I don't have a man in my life anymore." Maybe you don't today, but who says you won't have one tomorrow? I've seen it happen time and again, when it was least expected—a woman stops all sexual activity after her husband dies, and then later meets a man who awakens her, and she finds she has a greater sex drive than ever before.

One couple I was seeing is a good example of that. From what the husband said, the woman was very passionate, had a tremendous amount of sexual responsiveness. I knew this was her second marriage, and when I talked to her I said, "You must have been a terrific partner the first time around." To my great surprise, she said, "No, not really. This is something new to me." She had been married for twenty-nine years before, and for the last ten years her husband was quite sick. After the first husband died, she threw herself into sports—golf, tennis, swimming—and pretty much put sex out of her life. But after she remarried, her whole attitude changed. "I never dreamed sex could be so much fun," she said. "I don't think I ever had an orgasm with my first husband, but now I have them all the time. Sometimes more than one, in fact."

It happens. You meet the right person, the sparks fly, and

there is something that was never there before. That's why you should never let yourself lose interest, because you never know.

Another really major cause of loss of interest in sex is a lack of communication between the partners. Lack of communication is at the root of many of the problems we have in everyday life, so it's no surprise to find that it affects sex, too. It's not at all unusual for a couple to have less and less in common as they grow older. You can probably guess that the divorce rate is highest in the first couple of years of marriage, but did you know that the next highest time is after twenty-five years? It might be useful to look at some of the reasons for that.

Those are people who have never really gotten along throughout their married life, perhaps bickered constantly, never had too much in common, just sort of managed an existence with each other. But the man is struggling to get his career underway, the kids are being born and raised, and the couple has outside interests they can look to. The man can throw his energy into his work, and the woman can throw her energy into the house and into the kids, or perhaps into her own career or volunteer work and hobbies. That can be enough to keep them from really focusing on their problems as a married couple.

Then the kids are grown up; the man is a little more set in his career and begins to relax a little. Maybe the woman starts to think, "I've spent a lifetime being a housewife and mother. I've always been interested in art (or music or literature), I've always wanted to go back to school and finish my education."

At that point, they are likely to take the first good look at each other they have taken in a long time . . . and not like what they see at all. That's when they might decide to see if they can find something better out of life, and they get a divorce. Could the relationship have been saved? Yes, it might have been—if the couple had been made aware of their lack of communication early enough and had sought counseling to do something about it. Unfortunately, this kind of problem gets worse the longer it goes untreated. Even then, the counselor may find that the situation is beyond fixing and may recommend that a divorce is the best course.

* * *

The difference in the way men and women age sexually is another area ripe for misunderstanding. A man hits his sexual peak in his teens—he's capable of one ejaculation after another, with almost no recovery time needed. Then from the mid-twenties to about fifty there is a gradual slowdown. The slowdown continues after fifty, but here there is a difference among different men. If you were vigorous sexually before fifty, you aren't going to slow down as much afterward as you would if you were not vigorous. In other words if you had a vigorous sex life when you were young, you are going to be able to maintain that same vigorous sex life when you are older, but at a slower pace.

A woman, on the other hand, doesn't hit her sexual peak until her thirties and early forties. Not only that, the decline, when it comes, is very slow. A woman who is multi-orgasmic in her youth can remain multi-orgasmic all her life.

Here's a typical problem: the man gets older and his sexual vigor decreases, but the woman becomes more vigorous, in part, perhaps because she has been released from the fear of having children. And, unfortunately, he doesn't know how to accommodate her. He doesn't know what to do to help her out. He slows down and her needs stay pretty level for a long time. However, the fact that this happens isn't really in itself the problem. Those changes are going to take place no matter what they do, simply because that's how nature works. No, the problem is that they don't talk to each other about it, and they don't make the needed adjustments. They have to make adjustments, and in order to be able to do that they have to communicate.

I'll be talking about how to deal with that kind of problem later. Right now, I just want you to realize why you might find yourself becoming unresponsive if your partner's vigor diminishes and you're afraid to talk to him about it.

I'd like to go back to something I told you about earlier—the fact that a man does not have to ejaculate every time he has sex. If you understand and accept the fact that he is getting pleasure from the act whether he ejaculates or not, you can avoid a lot of conflict between you.

Suppose he can only manage one ejaculation per week, but you want to have sex three times a week. Well, if you realize that he doesn't need to ejaculate, then he can satisfy you all three times. That point is important enough to dwell on a little more. A man can be a good sexual partner without ejaculating—*and you have not failed him if he doesn't.*

It must have occurred to you by now that nothing has been said in this chapter about orgasms. I don't want you to get the idea that not having an orgasm is the same as not responding sexually. Nothing could be further from the truth. The fact is, most women who don't have orgasms *do* respond sexually. They love the petting, love the attention, love the playing and the stimulation—but they never get past the plateau stage, because something holds them back from letting go, from carrying the feeling all the way to orgasm.

It's almost as if the sexual response gets stuck, isn't it? That's about what does happen, in fact. Many women will allow themselves to be stimulated sexually up to a certain point, and then for one reason or another they will turn it off. Sometimes the cutoff is as definite as throwing a switch.

One of my women patients masturbates regularly; yet she has never had an orgasm. Why? Because as soon as she reaches a certain level, she stops cold. I was curious about that, because it is so different from the way a man would approach the same situation. Unless he is interrupted, there is no way a man is going to stop masturbating before he has an orgasm.

It turned out that the woman was embarrassed about what she was doing. She was afraid to let herself go completely enough to have an orgasm. If she was unable to relax enough to have an orgasm by herself, you can imagine how difficult it would be for her to do it with a partner. Sexual feelings are incredibly complex, and just because they are among the most natural and instinctive of our feelings doesn't make them any less so.

Maybe you are not having orgasms, but you are happy with your sex life the way it is. Then you don't have a problem, and what I'm going to talk about now doesn't really apply to you. But you might as well read it, anyway—you never know, you might change your mind. On the other hand, maybe you don't have orgasms and you're unhappy about it—you feel there's something missing. You're the one I want to talk to right now.

How did you get that way? Was it because you had a partner who didn't know how, or who didn't take enough time to bring you to orgasm? Was it because your partner was a premature ejaculator? Was there a lack of communication between you and your partner which made it impossible for you to tell him your needs? Was it because you felt it was his duty to make you orgasmic? Did you lie there all the time wondering if he was going to last long enough to bring you to orgasm?

Well, you are the one responsible for your own orgasm, you know. If you can't communicate with him and tell him how to bring you to satisfaction, how is he going to know?

How do you feel about your partner? Are you compatible, or does there always seem to be some source of irritation between you? Do you see eye to eye on things, or do you disagree a lot? How do you feel about your partner physically? If you can't stand to be touched by him, there is no way he is going to be able to bring you to orgasm.

The way you feel about your partner is important, but so is the way you feel about yourself. For example, are you happy with yourself physically? If you're not, you can't let yourself go sexually.

Those things could apply whether you've never had an orgasm in your life or you used to have them and don't have them now. A fairly common experience is that of a woman who used to have orgasms regularly, but has stopped having them for one reason or another. That's what we call a secondary sexual dysfunction, like the problem of secondary impotence in men.

There are a lot of reasons for secondary problems. A big one is depression. Depression can happen to anyone, and can be severe enough to stop even the most responsive of women cold. The loss of a loved one—a spouse, a member of your family, a close friend, even a pet—can make you lose your ability to reach orgasm. The realization that you are getting older, and with it the fear that you are losing your femininity, are also important factors.

Let's not forget social pressures. Worry about the opinions of others might make you feel funny about the fact that you're trying to be active sexually. If you feel funny about them, you can't relax.

There are also some physical and medical reasons you might lose your ability to have orgasm, but we'll talk about that later.

What do you need to have an orgasm? Basically, you need three things: 1) you must be properly stimulated; 2) you must be in the kind of surroundings that leave you sufficiently relaxed; and 3) you must have *no* orgasmic inhibitions—that is, you can't be afraid to show your sexual appetites.

Does a lot of that sound familiar? It should. You've heard much of it before, in one form or another. Although not being able to respond sexually and not being able to reach orgasm are two different problems, the causes are often the same.

I know I've given you a lot of causes for a lot of sexual problems, but don't let that discourage you. The very fact that we know what causes the problems means there is something that can be done about them. And if you have any of these problems yourself, that's one of the reasons you're reading this book—to find out what to do about them.

Chapter 6:
MEN AND MASTURBATION

I don't know how masturbation ever got to be thought of as "self abuse." That's about as far from the truth as I can imagine. On the contrary, masturbation is a completely natural instinct, as natural as laughing or crawling. The minute a baby can coordinate his hands, he goes right for the place where he gets pleasure, and that's his sex organs. You get a pretty good idea of how natural it is when you consider that a baby doesn't have to be taught to touch himself, but he does have to be taught *not* to touch himself. And, unfortunately, he is.

An important thing to remember about masturbation is that it's really the first sexual experience a man has, and nearly every man has had his first orgasm by self-manipulation. A visitor from another planet, confronted with that evidence, would have to conclude that masturbation is one of the best things we earthlings have going for us. But, as you well know, sadly that's not the way we think.

Is there any one of you who has not heard at least one horrible thing that is sure to happen to you if you masturbate? If you're like most men, you've heard a lot more than one of those stories. For example, you may have heard that you would become feeble-minded, that hair would grow on the palms of your hands and you would get warts. So I've got a question for you. Do you remember when you heard all those stories? That's right—when you were a kid. Considering the audience

I'm writing for, that was probably forty or more years ago. What have you been doing all this time? Among other things, you have probably been masturbating.

How do I know that? Easy. It's become common knowledge in the field of human sexuality that 95 percent of all men have masturbated. The other 5 percent either have something physically wrong with them that has kept them from masturbating, or they lie about it. I'm sure that if you examine yourself carefully, you won't find any symptoms of those horrible things you were warned about so seriously.

Well, maybe you never believed those myths and the others like them. But there might be other beliefs about masturbation that aren't as easy for you to shake. One common belief is that if you masturbate too much when you are young, you won't have anything left when you are older. That is absolute nonsense! It's every bit as much of a myth as the one about hair on your palms. You are not born with only a certain potential number of ejaculations and no more. There's no limit. There's always more where the last one came from. That's why there's no need to worry about having "wasted" them when you were young. In fact, the worst thing a man can do as far as maintaining his sexual vigor through his older years is concerned is to ration himself when he's young. All that does is get the body used to functioning at a slower pace. Have you ever noticed that in a store, the fast-moving items are restocked quicker than the slow-moving ones? That's because the demand creates the supply. It works kind of the same way with your body, too. Contrary to what the myth says, the more you use it, the better off you are.

I've mentioned several times before that everything about an older man's sex life slows down, and that the slowdown can trigger a lot of anxieties. One of those anxieties is likely to be about his masturbation in the past.

I have a patient now who's in his early fifties. He lives with an elderly aunt. Both of them are very neurotic. It wasn't easy to drag a medical history out of him, but one thing I did find out—for the previous ten years he had avoided any contact with women at all. During the week he always came right home from work to his aunt, and on a weekend his only pleasure was to sit in a bar and have a few drinks with some friends.

He didn't have a sexual experience with a woman until he was in his late thirties, and that was a resounding failure. He didn't know it was something that should be taken in stride, and he took the failure to mean he was no good with women, that the only kind of sexual activity he could be any good at was masturbation. He needed the sexual release, so he continued to masturbate. But the more he masturbated, the more he worried about it. The next thing that happened was he began to believe that all the masturbating he had done since he was a kid was affecting his mind.

He was afraid he was going insane, that he was becoming feeble-minded. He lost interest in his work, and he began to withdraw from the only social contacts he still allowed himself. He came to see me frequently and he was constantly asking me, "Do you think I'm going insane?" and "Will I end up in an institution?" Every time I suggested psychotherapy he got angry, because to his mind that reinforced his feeling that I thought he was insane. The last I heard, he had become a total recluse.

That is an extreme example of someone who was taught the wrong things about masturbation and unfortunately believed them.

When you take the myths and then add the attitudes of parents, church, society and even some medical men, it's no wonder masturbation has gotten such a bad name. Those myths and those attitudes have caused a lot of grief, because they make people feel guilty about doing something that is natural and perfectly harmless as well.

I'd like to give you an example of the kind of thinking that caused those myths and attitudes. In 1926, a doctor named Winfield Scott Hall published a book entitled, "The Intimate Life." The subtitle set out the purpose of the book in no uncertain terms— "Plain talks to parents and young people establishing a home."

Just in case any reader didn't know who the author was, or wondered about his qualifications to write on such an important subject, here's how he was identified on the title page:

"By Winfield Scott Hall, M.S., M.D., Ph.D., Professor Emeritus of the Medical Faculty, Northwestern University; Director, Bureau of Public Health, Board of Christian Education, Presbyterian Church, U.S.A.; Volunteer Medical Service, U.S. Public Health Service, during World War; Exchange Professor, Universitie Internationale, Brussels, Belgium; President, Child Conservation League of America; Author of 'Manual of Experimental Physiology, Nutrition and Dietetics,' 'Biology, Physiology and Sociology of Reproduction,' 'Sexual Knowledge,' 'Father and Daughter,' 'Father and Son, Chums,' 'From Youth into Manhood,' and Leading Authority on Social Hygiene."

Whew!

The average person at the time would have had a lot of difficulty arguing against the opinions of such an authority figure. And I'm sure the man was well known and highly respected in his day. Well, here's what this "Leading Authority on Social Hygiene" had to say about masturbation:

"The habit (masturbation) is easily acquired by boys during their preadolescent period. A boy may be led into the habit by a vulgar-minded older boy, or by a low-minded servant, or he may acquire the habit through some incident of his personal, private life and not influenced by anyone else.

"So many boys get into this habit that no boy may safely be left uninstructed; he should be told by his father or by some trusted man teacher or other leader of boys. In one of these ways he should learn of the harm that comes from handling the sex organs—exciting and irritating them so their work is disturbed.

"If a boy knows what harm self-abuse will do to him, he is quite sure to quit the habit if he has already acquired it; or if he has not gotten into the habit he is effectively guarded against it.

"Boys who have been circumcised are far less likely to get the habit of self-abuse than are boys who have not been circumcised.

"As a rule all that a small boy needs to help him break the habit of self-abuse is to have the matter clearly explained to him and to know that boys who are addicted to that habit do not develop into as fine, big, strong men as those who keep free from the habit. Explain to the boy that self-abuse is an unclean, unmanly habit. Explain also that it is important to keep his mind clean and free from vulgar thoughts."

See what I mean?

Premature ejaculation is the second most common form of sexual dysfunction in the male, and it is one of the unfortunate results of those attitudes. If you happen to come from a society where it was frowned upon—and most of our elderly population does—well, parents certainly didn't say, "Go ahead and masturbate." So it was always done secretly. It was done secretly and fast, because you didn't know when Mom or Dad might come along and catch you at it. Staying too long in the bathroom was a good way to arouse parental suspicion. It had to be gotten over in a hurry.

From some of the things my buddies told me, I knew that some parents were a lot tougher about it than others. For example, my folks never told me not to masturbate—of course, I never asked permission, either. The subject just wasn't discussed, so I had to go by instinct, and my instinct told me masturbation was something they didn't consider very nice. So I did it in secret. I assumed they wouldn't like it, and I had no desire to test my assumption at first hand.

However, one of my patients knew exactly how his mother felt about it. The way he tells it, she was convinced that masturbation was one of the most horrible sins possible for a human being to commit. When he was a teenager, the bathroom door could be opened from the outside even when it was locked. And that's what his mother did. She kept a sharp eye out for suspicious signs, and when she thought something fishy was going on, she flew into action like an avenging angel. Masturbation was a frantic, tense thing for him, and very rarely pleasurable. He never knew when he would be sitting on the toilet and suddenly see the door fly open. She caught him in the act quite a few times, and punishment always followed. The punishment was usually having a privilege taken away.

Did he ever stop masturbating because of that treatment? No, he didn't. What did happen was he became one of the worst cases of premature ejaculation I'd ever known. All he had to do was touch his penis to his wife's genital areas, and he would come. He was rarely able to manage full penetration before it happened, and if he did he never lasted past the first or second stroke. He went into therapy, finally, to get himself straightened out. After he got his premature ejaculation problem resolved, it still took awhile before he was able to relax and get real pleasure from sex.

The problems of an older man are different, however, especially the older man who is married. The big question for someone who is married is, "Why are *you* masturbating?" The obvious attitude is that there is something wrong with masturbating if you are married and have a sexual partner. Well, that's another myth. Masturbation is a natural instinct, and there's nothing wrong with it, whether you have a partner or not.

It's easy for me to say it's okay for a married man to masturbate, but that's not always so easy to accept, especially by the wife involved. Many wives are puzzled, insulted, and often greatly angered when it happens. The immediate reaction seems to be to blame themselves for something. Often the fact that her husband masturbates makes the wife feel guilty. She doesn't know what she feels guilty about—she just knows she feels guilty.

Very often I'm confronted with a woman who will come into my office and say, "Doctor, I don't know what's wrong with me. Goodness knows our sex life has slowed down, but when we do it, it is pleasurable. So here I am lying alongside of him, and I find him masturbating. Is there something wrong with me, or is there something wrong with my husband?"

The answer is neither. Masturbation is a natural habit that has gone on for years and years, and will go on for years and years. There is absolutely nothing wrong with either a man *or* a woman masturbating even when there is an available partner. The fact is, men *do* masturbate after marriage, and very often for reasons that have nothing to do with how good the marriage is. A man may masturbate because his wife is sick and can't have intercourse, or maybe because she is out of town for a while. You know, a lot of married men masturbate just because it feels good and they like it.

That's perfectly all right. The only time there might be a

problem about a married man masturbating is if he is doing that *instead* of trying to satisfy his wife. By that I mean if he is using masturbation as a means of wearing himself out physically so he can avoid having intercourse with his wife. But if his wife is satisfied, why shouldn't he masturbate if he wants to?

Actually, the man who can masturbate is very lucky. For instance, it's much easier to treat a man for impotence if he can masturbate. It's also a means of diagnosis, because a man who can masturbate with either a partial or full erection is not a totally impotent man.

The whole problem is very much like the wet dream at night. Even though it slows down as you get older, it can still happen. Again, it's a natural thing. You have a fantasy in your sleep and you have a wet dream. When that happens, a lot of men chastise themselves because they feel they are wasting it. They know things have slowed down for them, and maybe they are even aware that their partners might be feeling a little deprived—and there they are, having an ejaculation in their sleep, throwing it away. But wet dreams are not something you can control, and you shouldn't feel guilty about them.

You might think, "Why didn't I do it when I could do some good for both of us?" That's the worst thing about having a wet dream—and about masturbating as well—the thought that you're wasting an opportunity for helping out a situation that has slowed down. What I hope I can make all of you understand is that it isn't wrong to masturbate, especially as you get older. You get an urge and you want to satisfy it. Masturbation has many uses. First of all, it provides an outlet for sexual tension when no other form of release is available. To put that in plainer terms, it can keep you from climbing the wall when you get sexually frustrated.

Masturbating will keep you vigorous sexually, because it is another way for you to use your sex organs and keep your tissues vital. Masturbation is also very useful as a means of therapy, as a way to teach a man how to enjoy and respond to the feelings of reaching an orgasm. It's also used to teach a man how to break down his sexual inhibitions. As a matter of fact, there's a heightened feeling of excitement from masturbating that you don't get from intercourse.

Both men and women will tell you that masturbation gives them a more intense and exciting orgasm than they get from intercourse. Masturbation isn't as satisfying emotionally—the affection, warmth, and tenderness aren't there—but the excitement is higher. That figures, because after all, who knows where you are most sensitive and most easily stimulated better than you? For another thing, you have more of a chance to have fantasies if you are masturbating. Not only that, you can do it without feeling guilty about it. You can bring out any fantasy in the world. You can masturbate with any movie star or secret love of yours in your mind. And nobody will criticize you for it, because nobody can know what you are thinking.

A fantasy while you are having intercourse with a partner can be tricky, though. At the very least, it can make you feel rude. You feel as if you are doing your partner an injustice. Here you are, making love, and all of a sudden you feel yourself thinking of Hedy Lamarr. That can be an embarrassing realization. Sometimes when you're in an intimate situation with a woman, you get the feeling she can read your mind.

That reminds me of the story of the husband and wife who were making love and were both trying very hard to come to a satisfactory orgasm, but without any success. Finally the woman said to her husband, "What's the matter, can't you think of anyone, either?"

I'd like to reassure you about something at this point. You might feel guilty having a fantasy while you are making love to your mate, but believe me, you shouldn't. It's a very common thing to do. And don't think it's something that happens because a person finds his or her sex partner unattractive. Some of the youngest, most attractive couples I know admit to having fantasies about other people from time to time. There's no way that fantasizing like this is going to hurt your partner. And it's an easy way to put a little variety and fun in your life.

No matter what parents, the church, or society in general say about masturbation, it's a healthy natural function. And when something goes wrong with a man sexually, masturbation may be one of the methods used in the treatment. As far as the religious attitude goes, you might be interested in some remarks made by a young priest who was taking part in a panel discussion with me. I was pleased—and I have to admit, somewhat surprised—at the way he handled the question about whether masturbation is a sin or not.

The priest was asked by a member of the audience, "Father, how do you feel about masturbation? Does the church still consider it sinful?" And the priest answered, "What does God want of His children? He wants His children to be happy; He wants His children to be healthy. We've learned enough today about sexual physiology to know that a human being is a sexual being and needs release from sexual tensions. A man might inhibit his sexual impulses and then find that he can't forget them entirely or abstain without worry. He finds himself wanting to masturbate, but he doesn't, because he thinks it's wrong.

"That kind of emotional strain is really enough to make someone sick. He goes to the doctor with complaints generally psychosomatic, and most often related to the pelvic area, back, and legs. I'm sure the Lord wouldn't want him to be sick, and if suppressing normal sexual release makes a man sick—I don't think that would be God's intent."

I can't think of anything I could say that would improve on that statement.

Does aging affect masturbation? Sure it does, and in the same way it affects intercourse. The same things happen to you when you masturbate now as they did when you were young, but now they happen slower. To get more specific about it, if you're an older man, it's going to take a longer time to reach the excitement stage. When you get an erection, it's not going to be as firm as it once was. And when you do ejaculate, you'll have a very rapid resolution and a much longer period before you can attain another erection.

However, you can still do what I told you was possible to do with intercourse. After all, if it's not necessary for you to ejaculate during intercourse, why should it be necessary during masturbation? You can bring yourself to the plateau level, let the excitement subside—and then do it all over again. In fact, you could go on for hours like that if you wanted to.

To sum it up, masturbation is a very nice form of excitement, and it's a perfectly harmless means of having some fun and relieving sexual tension.

And there's absolutely nothing wrong with it!

Chapter 7:
WOMEN AND MASTURBATION

If a man tells me that he has never masturbated in his life, I would agree that he either has something physically wrong with him or he is lying. But if a woman says she has never masturbated, I'll believe her. Why? Because although almost all men masturbate (95 percent, as I've said before), that's not true of women.

Only about 65 percent of women masturbate. I'd like to point out right now that the 35 percent who do not masturbate are not necessarily women with sexual problems. Of course, some of them do have problems, but by no means all of them.

The question that seems to leap to mind at this point is, if men and women are both sexual beings—and they are—why don't as many women masturbate as men? I could just say that men and women are different, and leave it at that, but it wouldn't be a very helpful answer.

One reason a woman might not masturbate is that she can accommodate to denying herself sexually a lot more easily than a man can. She can adjust to not being excited, probably because she has been taught to associate sex so closely with emotional involvement. Society may have looked the other way when a man gave in to his "animal urges," but woe betide the woman who had sex for that reason. It has been my experience that people tended to be much kinder, more forgiving to a woman who was emotionally carried away, who was "swept off her feet." But if she gave in to plain everyday "animal lust," she was an outcast, a loose woman, a slut.

So, you see, where a man was conditioned to think of sex as a response to a physical need, a woman was taught to think of it as something she did because she was carried away by love and emotion and deep feeling for the man she was with.

That's why it's easier for her to give up sexual pleasure as a physical thing—she just wasn't taught to think of it as simply a physical thing, so oftentimes she really isn't as strongly aware that she is giving something up.

It's only been comparatively recently that many of those attitudes have begun to change, and believe me, they've got a long way to go before they change completely.

I've talked about sex being considered a duty, rather than a pleasure. That also shows an emotional, rather than a physical attitude toward sex.

Another aspect of this whole issue of women's attitudes is that a lot of women have the idea that their sex organs are somehow messy and unpleasant. That feeling is something that goes back to a woman's early training. For example, when she menstruates, she's very aware that she's bleeding from her vagina. I'll bet when most of you women were younger, you were made to feel ashamed because you weren't supposed to go swimming on certain days of the month. That's not true now (about the swimming or the attitude!), but it used to be.

A lot of myths have grown up around menstruation, and most of them are neither nice nor true at all. For example, there's a belief that a woman should not go near a plant while she is having her period because the plant will die. That myth and a lot of others are not only quite crazy, they are downright insulting. If they get repeated often enough, they can't help but have an effect on a woman.

There are even religious taboos surrounding menstruation. It's in the Old Testament that a woman was considered unclean from the time she started menstruating until a week afterward, when she took a ritual bath. Intercourse was totally forbidden during that time, until she was "cleansed" by the bath. That law is still observed by many Jews to this day.

Another thing that doesn't help is the general tendency to call menstruation by some euphemism. "I'm having my sick days," is one; "It's that time of the month," "My little friend is here," are others. The most common reference of all, I think, is "The Curse." You'll notice that most of those names are sarcastic or downright hostile, and it's not too hard to believe that a woman could transfer the hostility to the organ itself. However, attitudes about menstruation are changing. For one thing, modern methods of hygiene and sanitary protection have made it possible for women to participate in virtually all the activities they enjoy when they are not menstruating. Teaching about menstruation has also become more enlightened, and women are now being taught to think of it as the natural function of a healthy body and not as something onerous.

Sexual excitement, as you know, causes lubrication of the vagina, and that can bring another kind of problem. A young patient of mine told me of her experience. "When I was first dating and began necking and petting," she said, "I would come home and my underwear would smell different. Not an unpleasant odor, but a characteristic one that was usually only present at those times. I finally figured out that I had gotten wet down there from excitement, and my panties had also gotten damp from it."

It's surprising how even women who are very knowledgeable sexually sometimes don't make that connection. The thing is, you don't lubricate because you're about to have intercourse; you lubricate because you're sexually excited. But a woman who doesn't realize that, or who simply doesn't think of it, is going to see it as just another mess. Add to that the fact that when you urinate it comes from somewhere in there, and it's easy to see how the idea of the vagina being something involving unknown, mysterious discharges—and therefore because of lack of knowledge, possibly unpleasant—has been so deeply implanted.

Women used to be told, generally, "Don't touch, it isn't

nice." With that kind of conditioning, all you think about is that it gets wet and sloppy, it's near where the urine comes out, and it gets sticky when you get excited. With this kind of misinformation, no wonder many women have a bad attitude toward their own bodies and its normal functions.

Many women consider semen unclean, and if a man ejaculates into the vagina, that just makes another mess. I know a lot of women who run to the bathroom immediately after intercourse for a douche so they can feel clean again. One of my male patients told me about a woman he had dated who took that kind of fastidiousness one step further. They were about to make love, and he asked her if he needed to use a condom. She said, "No, that's all right, but don't come in me." He thought she had misunderstood him, so he questioned her again. She was on the Pill, but she just didn't want the mess.

I firmly believe that if women were taught, "Touch it because it's a nice part of your body and it feels good," they wouldn't think twice about any mess.

In the previous chapter, I talked about men masturbating, which all you women who read it will know all about. The rest of you women—the ones who haven't read that chapter yet, I want you to do it now! You know why—the more you learn about your partner, the more you are going to be able to understand yourself. Anyway, when men masturbate, one of the biggest problems they have is with guilt. And believe me, you don't have to get into extreme cases before that guilt is very, very heavy. When you consider how much more lenient the upbringing of most males is in our society, then imagine the massive guilt feelings women must have after they have been taught from childhood on—don't touch.

If a baby boy is caught playing with himself, the parents might just laugh about it. They won't tell him to go ahead and do it, but they laugh about it. They may even give him the impression that they think it's cute. At that age, at least, punishment or serious disapproval is fairly rare. On the other hand, God forbid a parent should catch a little girl doing the same thing. For some reason, society has decreed that her action is not cute at all. So instead of a laugh, the little girl is likely to earn herself a slap on the hand and the warning she will come to know so well, "Don't touch that!"

And that is how attitudes are formed. The little girl does some perfectly natural and healthy exploring of her body and is immediately punished for it. Not only that, she finds out that her sex organs are considered dirty. All of this at a very impressionable age. Is it any wonder that such a little girl is going to grow up not believing she's got something beautiful down there? That's why if a woman does masturbate, she doesn't think of it as something good she's doing for a nice part of her body, she usually thinks of it as something really shameful. A boy is likely to talk about masturbating quite openly, but a girl or a woman will not. She just won't discuss it. She hides her secret.

Nowadays, sexual encounters are generally a lot more casual than they used to be. But the older woman of today grew up having an emotional involvement with a man she had sex with. For men, on the other hand, sex has always been triggered by physical excitement—if he sees a sexy picture or gets the feel of a woman's body sitting next to him, that's often all he needs. But the woman wouldn't get excited unless she had some kind of emotional feeling for the man. It's interesting to note, by the way, that an *older* man—because he can't be so easily aroused—also attaches more importance to the emotional aspects of the relationship.

Over the years I have taught my residents how to spot the signs of women who are having sexual problems. If their complaints are related to the general pelvic area, such as persistent vague pain in the lower abdomen, backaches, tiredness, a dragged-out, heavy feeling in the legs, persistent and frequent urination and so forth, all of which are not confirmed by positive physical findings of disease, that's usually the tipoff. When I spot those signs, I casually ask, "How about your sex life?" If they are widows, I ask them, "Do you ever think about sex? Are you still interested in sex? Do you miss it? Do you fantasize? Do you masturbate?"

Some of them will say, "Oh, doctor, of course not! I never even think about it." Others will say, "Well, I do find that I may occasionally wake up in the middle of the night and find that I have been touching myself and feel somewhat excited, but I just pass it off as a dream." I see some women who deny they have any such ideas; yet when I examine them, I find scratch marks around the vulva near the vaginal opening. If I don't find any apparent reason for the itching—a rash or unusual dryness, say—I start to wonder why the woman is scratching. I might ask a few questions, but if she seems to be evasive, I usually don't press the issue. I'll give her a soothing lotion and something to calm her nerves and pursue the subject again the next time. Finally the woman will admit she does masturbate, or at least wants to, and then she begins to think she is doing something wrong and she shouldn't. So she scratches at herself in frustration.

Generally, I get all kinds of reactions to the question—embarrassment, anger, and guilt for having erotic desires at their age. They've been taught that older women just don't have erotic fantasies. And because it's something women don't discuss among themselves, they're really not aware other women do it.

Very few women will openly admit they masturbate for actual relief of tension. Many of them will say something like, "I never thought of it while my husband was alive, and for several years after he died, but all of a sudden I find myself getting ideas about sex that I haven't had in years." Whether those women actually masturbate or not, the guilt is usually there.

It's pretty well established that guilt—guilt about anything—causes emotional stress. As we in the medical profession well know, emotional stress very often produces physical symptoms, or psychosomatic symptoms. The symptoms could come from guilt about masturbation, or they could come from the stress caused by suppressing masturbation because of the feelings of guilt. It's strictly a no-win situation for anybody involved.

What some women do is find a kind of compromise—a compromise I'm not too happy about. What they do is excite themselves by having fantasies or by manipulating themselves until their organs get congested with blood from all that sexual stimulation. And that's it! In what can only be described as a futile try at having it both ways, they take the excitement that far, but they don't get any relief. They stop before they bring themselves to orgasm, because they want the pleasure, but they feel guilty about what they are doing. That is not healthy, not healthy at all. It often produces a condition known as chronic pelvic congestion because of that kind of repeated congestion without release. Not to mention the emotional damage that kind of fooling around can do. If they marry or begin a sexual relationship with a partner, they have established a behavior pattern that is almost certain to lead to a secondary sexual dysfunction. When they have intercourse, they will let themselves get as far as the plateau stage and then stop before reaching orgasm.

Those are some of the reasons women don't masturbate. How about some of the reasons why they *should*?

Masturbation not only relieves sexual tensions in a woman, it also helps slow down the aging process in her sex organs. A woman who continues sexual activity during her later years can help prevent her sexual organs from aging. That's true whether the sexual activity is intercourse or masturbation. The method makes no difference. Those women are not as often subject to senile vaginitis. They don't have the skin dryness around the external genitalia that produces cracking and itching. The woman who was multi-orgasmic in her youth can remain multi-orgasmic all her life by self-manipulation. Unlike a man, a woman can masturbate to orgasm as often as she wants to, because the recovery time is short for her.

There's a very popular concept in psychology today that deals with the problems people have in getting past the blocks that keep them from doing things they want to do. The treatment for that problem is to teach the people to give themselves permission, or to have some kind of an authority figure give them permission to do it. When I tell women who come into my office that it's all right to masturbate, many of them look very relieved, and I'm sure it solves many of their problems.

Take an adult woman who has never masturbated and has had a fairly satisfying marriage. Her husband dies, and after a while she begins to miss the sexual release. She has never masturbated, so she doesn't know what to do. She sits around feeling frustrated, and she worries about it, and finally she gets distress symptoms. That woman can be cured by teaching her to masturbate. It's perfectly normal for her to masturbate.

She never had any problems with the idea of her husband touching her and exciting her, but she can't bring herself to excite herself. The reason may not even be based on a religious or moral taboo, either. It's just something she never did, so it's a behavior pattern now. What I would try to do in her case is break that behavior pattern and teach her new behavior.

Sometimes clearing up the problem is as simple as giving her permission to masturbate, but not always. The treatment depends on how deep the problem is, and how long it has lasted. A serious disorder that has been around for a long time is not going to be cured by one word. It is going to take time and repetition.

A woman of sixty-seven came to see me with a complaint of persistent itching in the vaginal area. She was from a strict religious background. When I examined her, I couldn't find anything wrong. Now that puzzled the hell out of me, because her itching was really severe. With that kind of complaint, I expected to find all kinds of things—a rash, excessive dryness with scaling, maybe even pubic lice. But there was nothing. I gave her some lotion and sent her home. And she was back in a week with the same complaint. That's when it occurred to me that there might be a sexual problem. The other clue was that she was a widow.

So I said to her, "By the way, do you ever feel sexually inclined—like you want to touch yourself, like you want to excite yourself?" She said, "You know, that's a funny thing, doctor. I could care less when I was married whether I had intercourse or not. I don't remember that in my younger days I masturbated or touched myself. I just never thought about it. My husband's been dead about five years, and it never occurred to me until six months ago that I might have some sexual urges. Now I find I want to touch myself, I want to stimulate myself. I know it's wrong, so I don't do it."

I told her, "It's not wrong, it's perfectly all right. In fact, it's a good release for you." She told me, "I don't know, doctor, I'm not that kind of a person." Well, I didn't want to push the issue too hard, but I talked to her about it a bit more, and as she was leaving, I said casually, "If you decide to do it, I'd suggest using a little lubricant, so you don't irritate yourself." She didn't come back for several weeks, and when she did come back she was fine. The problem of the itching was gone.

The best thing about masturbation is that it's a good way to keep sexually active, especially if there is no sexual partner available. That's a real problem for an older woman. But just because a woman doesn't have a partner now doesn't mean she's going to be alone for the rest of her life. Who knows when she might find a man and want to get involved again. Well, if she doesn't masturbate, the aging process is going to take its toll.

But—if she continues to masturbate, she will slow the aging process down, and she will be able to function fully and comfortably when and if she meets somebody and wants to get sexually involved.

I know that for some of you, masturbation has always been abhorrent—something you cannot and must not do. If you feel that way, and you feel that way strongly, I will not urge you to masturbate, because for you to do so might just cause more serious problems. If you find masturbation too horrible to think about, for whatever reasons, then don't do it.

However, I strongly believe that masturbation is good for you. It's a healthy thing to do—providing you can accept it emotionally without shame or guilt.

Chapter 8:
ACHIEVING SEXUAL SATISFACTION

The most obvious question to ask at this point is, "What is sexual satisfaction?" Basically, it's anything that two people do for or with one another that pleases them. Does that sound pretty vague? Well, it was meant to be. You see, there is no one-size-fits-all definition of "sexual satisfaction."

After all, people are different. In fact, they are far more different from each other than they are alike. That's even true of you as an individual, you know. You don't always want the same things all the time, do you? Of course not! No matter how set you might be in your ways, from time to time you are going to want a change. Sexual satisfaction, like a lot of other things, depends on the individual. There's no way to make a definite rule, because what satisfies you might not satisfy your partner. Not to mention that what satisfies you today might bore you or turn you off tomorrow.

For some people, especially the age group I'm writing this book for, sexual satisfaction is a closeness, an intimacy and a loving affection between two people, without anything else at all. Other people would agree with the above, but would want to add a little petting and a little stroking—but stop short of actual intercourse.

For still others, sexual satisfaction runs the whole gamut—petting, stroking, affection, arousal, and then intercourse.

If a couple has reached the point where they are just as happy to abstain from bodily contact other than closeness, the verbal expression of satisfaction is enough for them.

Which reminds me of a story. One day, John was visiting his doctor for a routine checkup. Now, John and his wife, Maggie, were both in their eighties, and were obviously a very happily adjusted couple. The doctor had been curious about them for a long time—about their sex life, I mean—but he didn't know how to approach the subject. Finally, he asked, "John, do you satisfy Maggie?"

"Oh, yes, I satisfy her every night," said John.

"Every night?" asked the doctor.

"Oh, most every night," John replied.

"How do you satisfy her?" asked the astonished doctor.

"Well, I see that she's tucked in comfortably in bed, ask her if she needs a glass of water. I see that her teeth are put into the glass next to her bed, and I adjust her pillows. Then I say to her, 'Maggie, dear, are you satisfied?' and she says, 'Yes, honey, I'm satisfied.' "

So you see, almost anything can be a form of sexual satisfaction. It simply means that you and your partner engage in intimate contact with one another. That intimate contact can be physical, verbal—or even done by pantomime. You can do as much or as little as you wish. If you feel you have done enough, and you liked it, then you have achieved sexual satisfaction.

I said something about "intimate" contact, didn't I? How do you achieve that intimacy? Well, I can answer that question with one word—communication! We hear so much about the word communication. What does it mean, really?

Communication is simply the way you let each other know what you like or dislike. There are many ways of communicating your sexual needs and desires. You can do it by telling your partner, "I like this," or, "Don't do this, it's a little irritating." You can put your partner's hand where you want it to be, or you can move it away from where you don't want it to be. Sometimes just snuggling up close is all the communication you need.

Telling your partner you don't like something is not always easy, because a sexual encounter puts a person in a very vulnerable position emotionally. That's why it's important to be gentle with your partner, and even suggest something else that you know you will like, if possible. One thing *not* to do is say, "AAAAGH! That hurts! Don't do that!" The tone of voice you use, and the way your partner feels after you say it—those are the important things.

Many people get their sexual kicks from using vulgar four-letter words during the sex act. Or if they don't use the words themselves, they like to hear them. I get all kinds of reactions to that from my patients. Some of them like the practice, some are totally turned off by it, and some could care less.

I have a patient who has started dating again several months after his wife died, and he found one woman who seemed to be very responsive, someone who might be a really exciting sex partner. Well, she was. She was everything he could have dreamed about, but . . .

"But the more excited she got, the worse she swore, like an old-time sailor or something," he said. "That just turned me off. I stopped right then and there, in the middle. I just got off, that's all. I couldn't take it. She realized that, and she apologized. She told me she was sorry, she happened to be like that, and it was the only way she could come. I never called her again, never went out with her again."

That was something he'd never encountered before. His wife had never done it, nor had any of the women he dated after she died. Fortunately, he was only dating her, and he was able to literally walk away from the situation. Imagine the problem he would have had with it—considering how strongly he felt—if he had married her and not found out about her language habit until after the ceremony.

I've had other patients who have had exactly that happen to them. What do they do about it? Very often, they come to me and complain. The first thing I do when they come to me with the problem is talk to the one who likes to use the rough language. I might say, "Obviously, this is the way you get satisfaction, but you've got to realize that the four-letter words are making it difficult, if not impossible for your partner to be satisfied. After all, your goal in having sex is for both of you to get satisfaction." Then I suggest a compromise—finding words that are not as offensive to the one partner, but are still exciting to the other.

Asking the "talker" to give up the practice completely isn't realistic, because there's nothing actually wrong or harmful about it. In my experience, the best solution has been to just ask him or her to tone it down a little, to the point where it doesn't bother the partner.

How would you go about finding out what words are okay with your partner? Simple—you'd ask. It all comes down to communication again. Just ask your partner, "How do you like this word if I use it? Does that offend you?" You'll notice I haven't given you any examples. I'd rather not do that, because you're much more likely to find words you are comfortable with if you think of them yourself. In this case, I would strongly suggest you hold the discussions at times when you are not trying to make love.

With all this emphasis on communication, it sounds like I'm trying to turn every sexual encounter into a regular gabfest, doesn't it? No, that's not what I have in mind at all. But there does seem to be a prevalent attitude that sexual time is "quiet time." Somehow we've been brought up so we don't talk when we have sex. Where is it written we can't talk during sex?

I'm not saying you should talk during the actual sex act if you don't want to. You might find it so distracting you can't function, and that would defeat the purpose of the whole thing, wouldn't it? You might find that talking is a good way to begin, because it can be a nice way to ease into sexual activity. That's especially true as you get older and you need more time for your body to respond. You might be very pleasantly surprised at how much relaxed, intimate conversation can add to the pleasures of stroking and caressing. You might find it a good time to talk about your sexual likes and dislikes, or you might find it the worst time in the world to talk about those things.

Remember, I told you before how emotionally vulnerable people are at that time, so if you do talk about your likes and dislikes, it's a good idea to be careful what you say. You can talk about your sexual preferences before the act, while you're doing it, or after you've finished. The main thing is—talk about them!

Once you start to communicate and tell each other what you want and don't want, you're going to find out something really interesting about your sexual relationship. You're going to find out that you and your partner don't always want to do the same thing at the same time—and you might even find you want to do things your partner doesn't want to do anytime. It can work the other way, too. Your partner might ask you to do something *you* dislike.

I'd like to warn you about something right now. Don't let yourself fall into the trap of assuming that if your partner says "no" to something you ask for, your request was unreasonable. Is it unreasonable to want oral sex? Is it unreasonable to want to try new positions for intercourse? Is it unreasonable for a woman with increased sexual vigor to ask for relief from a husband who can't match her vigor in his later years?

None of those things is unreasonable in itself. All of them, in fact, are common varieties of sexual expression. But because most people do have some different needs and desires, conflicts are going to arise. Very often, conflicts can be resolved by just airing them out. On the other hand, there are such things as unreasonable demands—one partner demanding or forcing a performance on the other. Sometimes a reasonable request can quickly turn into an unreasonable demand.

Let's see how that can work in actual practice. John wants oral sex, and he asks Mary to do it to him. It's a perfectly reasonable request, and Mary knows it is a perfectly reasonable request. But she doesn't want to do it. No big moral or psychological taboo—it's just something she doesn't particularly like doing. So she says no. Right now, you have a conflict, and the only way to resolve the conflict is to talk about it.

Well, they talk about it. And they talk about it. No matter how much they talk about it, Mary doesn't want to do it. This is the place where it gets a little tricky. Up till now, John's request was reasonable. But if he pushes it past this point and coerces or forces Mary to do something she doesn't want to do, then the demand is unreasonable.

There's no way to compromise, either. It's one of those situations that comes down to either you do or you don't. The only thing John can do at this point is get used to the idea that oral sex is not the only way to get satisfaction. There are plenty of other things he can do. In fact, if he doesn't do just that, the irritation over the situation could very easily become the starting point for a serious dysfunction in one or both of them.

It wouldn't be a bad idea at this point for you to stop and take the time to do a little thinking. Oh, yes, I have something specific in mind. I'd like you to think about what you like about sex. I'd like you to sit down and figure out what you like to do unto others, and what you would like others to do unto you. It's such an obvious idea I'm sure you think you've already done it. You probably haven't, though, so do it now.

You might think that discovering what you like is a matter of "I'll know it when I see it." Maybe it is, but you can save yourself a lot of time and energy, as well as a lot of frustration, if you think it out a little first. And, believe me, any efforts you make in that direction are going to be greatly appreciated by your partner. Guessing games don't make for the best kind of sexual relationship. I firmly believe you get more pleasure out of anything if you know and understand what you enjoy about it.

The most important thing about sex is enjoying it. And that's what makes it so wonderful—it's fun, it's easy to do, and . . . it's okay! Sex should be something you and your partner both enjoy. When you start to make the enjoyment part work, when you start having fun, that's when you'll experience real sexual satisfaction. You'll notice I didn't say, "Sexual satisfaction is when you are touched two inches to the left and an inch and a half down from your right shoulder blade," or anything else that specific.

Sexual satisfaction doesn't work that way. For you it might be kissing, it might be petting, it might be hugging—or it might be oral-genital sex or trying every possible kind of sexual gymnastics. What the fun actually consists of doesn't matter. The only thing that matters is what you do should be fun.

Sex should be something you're comfortable with. One of the big reasons people don't find sex satisfying is they are uncomfortable with it. Many of you find sex embarrassing to talk about, or even think about, because you've been conditioned to believe there's something not quite nice about it. Sex is something you do in private, quietly, and usually in the dark. You make sure nobody can see or hear what you are doing, and you don't discuss it with your friends or neighbors. I think most people are not really very proud of themselves for having sex.

How can you possibly enjoy something you're not comfortable with? The answer is, you can't. There's no way you can really enjoy something you aren't completely at ease with. A lot of problems come to the surface when one partner is comfortable with some specific thing and the other isn't. The only way to resolve the situation is for both of them to be comfortable.

I've had many patients come to me and say, "I can't relax and enjoy sex because I've got all these inhibitions I can't get rid of. I was taught it just isn't right to do some kinds of things." I can understand that. It's never easy to go against what you were taught, whether what you were taught was right or not. You're bound to feel funny about it. Maybe you're not aware of it, but feeling guilty about something is very often taking the easy way out. You're taking the easy way out because it's less trouble to feel guilty about what you're doing than to think about whether it really makes sense for you to feel guilty or not.

Do you really think it makes a lot of difference to anyone else what you do? And even if it does, how are they going to know—unless you tell them. Seems to me the solution to that problem is a simple one—don't tell them!

When I was dating before I married again, I took a woman to a movie. In spite of the fact that it was touted as the comedy hit of the year, the theatre happened to be almost empty. My date sat through the show in absolute silence, and I thought, "She's bored to death; she'll never want to go out with me again." Much to my surprise, as we left the theater, she said, "Thank you. That was the funniest thing I've seen in years." I thought she was either kidding me or being nice until she called up the following week and asked me if I'd like to see the same movie again. We went again, and this time we didn't go so early that we missed the crowds. There was an almost full house. Talk about a difference! My date laughed out loud until tears ran from her eyes.

You've all had the experience, I'm sure. Nobody likes to think he or she is the only one doing something. You don't like to be the only one laughing in a theatre. That's why they started putting laugh tracks on TV shows, by the way, so people would feel like they were laughing as part of an audience. That kind of thing happens with sex, too. Suppose you want oral sex, but you have the idea you're the only one in the world wants to do it. You're bound to feel guilty about it, aren't you. But then, what if you discover almost everybody wants the same thing? You'll feel a lot different about yourself.

The real value of the Kinsey Reports when they came out was not so much that they told us what kinds of sexual things people were doing, but that they told us how many people were doing them. The study made it known that what people had kept hidden from everybody else was not something they alone were doing. Then Masters and Johnson came along and explained how and why people were doing such things.

It's been said often enough that there are no new plots in fiction, and I would venture to say there are no new ways to have sex. Which means, whatever you are doing, you didn't invent it; and whatever you are doing, you aren't the only one.

One of the best things about sex, as far as I'm concerned, is that it can be so spontaneous. There's something about getting the urge and then being able to satisfy it right away that is tremendously exciting. "Wait a minute!" I can hear some of you saying, "At my age, how am I going to be spontaneous? Are you telling me I'm going to come home feeling a little sexy, pat my wife on the fanny, and the next thing you know we're on the floor together with our clothes strewn all over the living room? That might work for a twenty-year-old kid, but you keep telling me I'm slowing down."

Right! That kind of scene would be ridiculous at your age. But try this one on for size. Suppose you come home and your wife is in the shower, and you decide it might be fun to get in there with her, so you do. Then you spend a lot of time soaping each other, some more time rinsing each other off, and then even more time rubbing each other dry. Maybe you kind of drift over to the bed and continue what you've started at an easy, enjoyable pace. If that isn't spontaneity, I don't know what is! It may be spontaneity in slow motion, but is still spontaneity. What happens as you get older is, the spontaneity is as fast as it ever was—carrying it out is going to be slower.

Here's something I've mentioned several times before, but I think is worth repeating in this context: it is not necessary for an older man to ejaculate every time he has sex. Now, I'm not talking here about your physical needs or well-being. I'm talking about satisfaction. You don't need an orgasm to have sexual satisfaction. Figure it out for yourself. Which is going to be more satisfying: having an orgasm every time, whether you need one or not, and being out of action for three or four days; or having the orgasm only when your body says you really need it, and being able to come back about as often as you want to?

I've been asked many times what I think of the practice of faking an orgasm. I don't like it. You don't really give your partner any more or any less pleasure that way, and you may do some emotional damage. You might get away with it for a while, but it won't take long for your partner to catch on. It's not easy to keep on fooling someone you are intimate with. I think faking an orgasm is a form of deception, and I think deception does not belong in an intimate relationship.

So you don't have an orgasm, don't fret. Tell your partner you didn't, but that you still got pleasure from what you were doing, and that you are satisfied. The matter of satisfaction is the important point, after all, not the orgasm.

One of the things I mentioned earlier was how important it is for you to know what you like about sex, what turns you on. The reason for that is obvious. You are the expert on yourself. You are the one who knows best what your needs and desires are. And the only way your partner is going to know is if you tell him or her.

Don't assume your partner knows what you want. A newspaperman once told me a journalistic maxim I think applies perfectly here: "Never underestimate your reader's intelligence, but never overestimate his knowledge of a particular subject." You've got to give your partner credit for being intelligent, compassionate and sympathetic, but you've also got to give your partner information. And remember, giving people information is not putting them down—it's helping them to function better.

Telling somebody what you like is hard enough, but telling somebody what you *don't* like can be extremely difficult with a subject like sex. I've known people who would put up with all kinds of discomfort and even pain because they weren't able to ask their partners to stop something they didn't like.

Martha, a woman in her early sixties, is a good example of that. When her husband caressed her, he always made direct contact with her clitoris. "I'm very sensitive there, and after a couple of minutes I'm ready to scream with pain," she said.

"Well, why don't you?" I asked her.

"Oh, I couldn't do that. Paul would get angry at me if I said anything to him about it."

"Let him get angry," I said. "Which is better for you in the long run—to have him angry for a while, or to fix once and for all a problem that is really bothering you, and can only get worse?" It took a lot more talking to convince her, but finally I did.

The point is, you should never tolerate anything you dislike, even if it means getting your partner angry. I think you'll find, though, you can usually manage to get your point across without upsetting your partner. It's perfectly all right for you to tell your partner a certain position or manner of caressing is uncomfortable or painful for you. Anyway, the chances are good that your partner won't resent it at all, but be happy for the chance to give you more pleasure.

Role playing is a terrific way to put some zip into your sex life. You have fantasies—everybody does—so why not act them out? Some of them might not be very easy to do, but you'll be surprised at how many will work that way. Make a game out of it, a kind of mini-adventure, a romp. For example, here's what one man I know did. He and his wife had both been big *Mission Impossible* fans when it was on TV. That's the show, you may remember, that always opened with the hero listening to a tape recording that gave him the details of his secret mission.

So one day my friend made sure he was home before his wife, and got everything ready. When she got home, almost the first thing she saw was their portable cassette recorder with a note on it. The note simply instructed her to push the "play" button. Well, what he had done was record complete instructions for a sexual "mission" which was designed to end in their mutual satisfaction. He even managed to put it in the kind of phrasing they used on the TV show.

She was delighted. She followed every one of his instructions to the letter, and it turned out to be one of the best times they ever had with each other sexually. "Setting the situation up and thinking about her reaction to it was almost as much fun as actually doing it," he said.

If you do things like that—make up games, allow yourself to be free, follow through and get caught up in the spirit of the thing, you can have a lot of fun. This is a good time in your life to be frivolous again. Don't ever think that just because you have reached a certain age, frivolity is beyond you. As long as you do it in the privacy of your own home, you can be as free and easy as you want.

You're very lucky if you happen to be retired. You have a lot more time to play. You don't have to wait until evening, when you come home from work. You can do it earlier in the day while you are still fresh.

All too often, people think they have to wait until something really serious is wrong with them before they can ask for help. For heaven's sake, come and talk to somebody if you aren't getting satisfaction from sex. Sex has been around for a long time, and you're not going to surprise a doctor—or embarrass him, either. Don't be afraid to ask directly about your problem. So many people come to me because they want to talk to me about their sexual problems, but what they wind up telling me is all about their aches and pains. The aches and pains might be real aches and pains, but they aren't the real problem. It's the sex that is the real problem.

I'd like to add that sexual satisfaction is not what your neighbors tell you it ought to be—it is not what the magazine articles and books tell you it ought to be. It is not even what some doctors tell you it ought to be. It is what you and your partner think it ought to be and feel that it is. And if what you feel is satisfactory to you, that is sexual satisfaction. Which, by the way, would include an affectionate relationship with a member of your own sex. It's easy to understand how older people might ease into such a relationship because of their loneliness and their need for the closeness of another human being. Their accepting of each other that way harms neither themselves nor anyone else.

Something as simple as a touch at the right time can be a completely satisfying experience. A friend of mine told me of just such an experience he had recently:

"I wanted to make love to my wife one night, and for some reason she couldn't or didn't want to. I tried rolling over and going to sleep, but I was restless because I was still turned on. So I decided to help myself out and masturbate. We are both comfortable with the idea of masturbation, because we do it so we won't put any sexual pressures on each other.

"Anyway, I proceeded to masturbate right alongside her in the bed while she continued to read. Just before I reached orgasm, I was vaguely aware that she had put down her book and was watching me. At the moment I came, she reached over and touched me affectionately on the cheek. She didn't feel she could make love to me that night, but she was right there to share my moment of pleasure with me. I felt very close to her then."

It's only when you feel you're missing something and you can't be convinced you are not missing something that I think you might need help. So I'll say again, the best place to start is with your family doctor, who knows you, and with whom you will be more comfortable talking.

Chapter 9:
WHAT IF YOU'VE BEEN SICK?

One of the first points I made in this book was that if you couldn't function sexually, the reason was probably in your head. I told you that nine out of ten cases of sexual dysfunction were psychological in origin. Well, that leaves one out of ten with a sexual problem that is purely physical. Those physical problems—or, as we call them, organic problems—could be happening to you now or they could happen to you at some other time. That's why I think it's important to discuss them.

Organic diseases can be bad enough by themselves, but to add insult to injury, any organic disease is very likely to affect you psychologically as well. Why? Because if you are sick, you worry, you have anxieties—and all those worries and anxieties are translated into fear. It should be no secret to you now that fear is probably the basic cause of most sexual dysfunctions. What kind of fear? Fear of performance, fear of being a failure, and indifference are good examples.

Short-term indifferences can happen to anyone. If you're under a lot of pressure at the office, for example, you can be completely indifferent to anything but your work problems for however long it takes to clear them up. That's not really something to worry about. The time you should start to worry is when you suddenly become indifferent to other things in your life. You don't enjoy your food as much anymore; you're not interested in TV; you don't particularly care to read a paper; you don't care if your grandchildren come to see you or not. Along with all that indifference, comes an indifference to sex, of course.

When someone who had been sexually functional becomes indifferent to sex and the indifference lasts for any length of time, you can be sure there is a sexual dysfunction, because sex is usually the last thing a person loses interest in. For example, if a man whose level of sexual activity was to have intercourse once a week starts making excuses and lets the activity dwindle to only once a month or less, that's an obvious sign of indifference. And that indifference can turn into a sexual dysfunction, which if allowed to continue will be very serious.

If all those things are going on, it's almost certain that the person involved is suffering from depression. You might wonder why I am discussing depression in a chapter about organic diseases. The reason is, although depression is not an organic disease, it works on the body in exactly the same way. Depression produces physical changes in the body just as organic disease does. There are changes in hormone secretion; there are changes in the ability to feel erotic sensations; there are changes in the ability to have an erection. While depression is not an organic disease, it is treated as one, and it must be cured before the sexual problem can be cured.

Is it possible to function sexually if you're depressed? Yes it is, in some cases. That depends on the depth of the depression. Depression can make you compulsive about sex, just as it makes some people compulsive about eating. You try to avoid thinking about your depression and feeling sorry for yourself, so you make yourself do things you wouldn't ordinarily do.

Generally, though, depression does retard sexual activity. Men can't get an erection, or if they can get one, they can't hold it. Women won't lubricate if they aren't interested. The difference is, a woman can lubricate herself with a water-soluble jelly. (Don't use Vaseline, because it will block any natural lubrication that might occur. The water-soluble jellies don't prevent natural lubrication.) She can then complete the sex act. She doesn't have an erection to worry about.

Depression is not something to fool around with, and it's not something to ignore. It has to be gotten out of the way before any other problems can be taken care of. The best thing you can do about depression is to go to your doctor, who will either help you himself or refer you to a good psychotherapist. The idea of doing that may bother you because you've heard stories of people who have been in therapy for years and years, and the end never seems to be in sight. I'm not asking you to sign up for life. All I'm suggesting is you see someone for an evaluation session or two. After one or two visits, the therapist will be able to tell you what kind of help you need.

Even though the odds strongly favor a sexual problem being psychological, the first thing I would do if you came to consult me would be to give you a complete physical examination. Why? I would want to rule out a physical cause right away, if I could. I would also want to know if your sex organs are healthy and functioning the way they should be.

We've talked about emotional and psychological needs before—but what do we need physically to have satisfactory sex? We need healthy sex organs, and the things that make them healthy are: 1) a good blood supply, 2) good muscle tone, and 3) a good hormone balance.

The blood supply is necessary to produce vasocongestion, which you will remember is the filling of your organs with the blood that makes them able to function the way they are supposed to. The male erection is an example. The erection is caused by the blood filling the tissues. In the woman, the blood supply congests the vaginal tissues and helps them produce lubrication. We still don't understand exactly how that works, but we do know the flow of blood causes the lubrication. The blood also makes the clitoris and the nipples of the breasts become erect.

When we talk about the nerve supply, we mean the nerves that stimulate the blood vessels to open and congest the tissues. The nerves produce the muscle tension that makes ejaculation possible for the male, and the vaginal contraction in a woman, during orgasm. The nerves also make the sensations we feel interesting enough to make our bodies react to them. You can think of your nerves as wires, carrying energy to your organs to make them function—just as electrical wires carry current to lamps and appliances in your home. If you have a weak nerve supply, it's like a sudden drop in electrical current. Your lights go dim, and your machines don't run as well as they are supposed to, because they're not getting enough energy.

Hormones are substances that are produced by the internal glands to regulate your bodily functions and keep everything in balance. The sexual hormones make your body function sexually, and they give you the desire to have sex.

You do almost everything better and enjoy it more when you are healthy. Why should sex be an exception? If you don't feel well, sex is usually the last thing you want to think about. When you're sick, you've got to expect a decline or even complete lack of interest in sex. That's a normal reaction, and it's going to happen—so don't start to worry if a cold or bout with the flu knocks the urge right out of you. If you leave it alone and get well, the urge should come right back.

I know all of you appreciate consideration and understanding when you are sick, so if your partner is the one who is ill, please be considerate if he or she is not interested in sex.

You respond to illness one way, I respond another. Some of you are hit hard by disease, others seem to breeze through a plague with hardly any sign that they are more than slightly off their feed. I've seen people in the hospital who are really seriously sick being caressed and fondled by a husband or wife and loving every minute of it. But in the next bed or down the hall there might be someone not nearly as sick who would climb the walls in agony from merely being touched.

The important thing to remember about illness is—don't worry. If you are worried about illness, if you are afraid you can't function, if you are afraid that having sex will aggravate your illness, you aren't going to be able to function sexually. To be able to enjoy sex, you have to be completely free to give vent to your emotions, without any restrictions.

You're probably starting to worry about illness in general. Don't. There isn't as much to be concerned about as you might think. Most illnesses only partially affect sexual functioning.

And even the more serious diseases—like severe diabetes, or certain liver diseases, cardio-vascular diseases (heart and blood vessels)—might only have a partial effect on sexual functioning. That's why I never assume that just because a person has a disease which tends to produce sexual dysfunction, that person is totally unable to function sexually.

I'm thinking of a couple who have been coming to see me for years. The woman is in her late sixties and he is in his early seventies. He's a diabetic, and the world's worst patient as far as following orders about insulin dosage and diet. No matter what I tell him, *he* decides how much insulin he wants to take. His idea of regulating his diet is: he eats what he likes and doesn't eat what he dislikes. His wife is constantly battling him: "Why don't you ever do what the doctor wants?"

One day in the course of a consultation in my office she said to me—right in front of him— "Do you know, this old man still has ideas?" And I said, "What do you mean, 'ideas?' " She told me, "He wants to behave like he did when he was young, and he can't."

He wanted to have intercourse, but because of his illness and the way he took care of himself, he couldn't. So I said to her, "What's wrong with having ideas? He still feels like he wants to be affectionate, and there's nothing wrong with that. He can still make you feel good, and by making you feel good he makes himself feel good. As long as he wants to do it, I see no reason you shouldn't let him."

I took advantage of the occasion to do some plain talking to him, too. I told him that not all diabetics are completely impotent, and if he took the trouble to control the disease, he might regain some of his sexual potency. He didn't change overnight, but after a while he began to take his insulin as directed, he ate what he was supposed to eat, and we finally got his blood sugar down to where it was relatively safe.

I don't think he ever did get back the ability to have erections, but the fact that he was taking care of himself removed the source of most of their fighting, and his wife was able to respond to his gestures of affection. They did seem a lot happier with each other.

I always figure it's worth a good try to treat the person.

Many times, there will be success. And even if the success is only partial, the person might be able to learn new ways of getting satisfaction. They might not be able to do exactly what they did before the illness, but they can learn to adjust to what they can do, and be happy with it.

I'm not really talking about simple illnesses, because they don't really affect your sexual ability. They might slow it down for a bit, and even stop it cold for a couple of days or a week or so—but being exceptionally busy can do the same thing. A simple illness is merely an interruption—not a problem. If you have a fever and you ache all over, you don't want to have sex. When the fever and the aching go away, the urge will probably come back.

What I want to talk about here are the debilitating illnesses and conditions—diseases like diabetes, arteriosclerosis, multiple sclerosis, strokes, and heart attacks. Other things that cause serious sexual problems are conditions that produce weakness, conditions that affect blood vessels, and painful conditions—such as arthritis, backaches, neuritis. By painful conditions I mean problems that allow you to function successfully, but hurt when you do so. Other painful conditions are certain diseases of the vagina such as senile vaginitis or vaginismus—or maybe scar tissue around the vagina due to surgical procedures that produces pain upon intercourse. Priapism is a male condition which falls in this category. The man who suffers from it has a perpetual erection, which can become quite painful over a long period of time.

There is also a disease in which a man's penis is bent or crooked. That might sound funny, but let me assure you, it's not. It's difficult for a man with this condition to insert the penis into a vagina because of the angle, and that can be painful and unpleasant.

Those are some of the things that nature does to you. How about some of the physical problems you can directly bring upon yourself? Drugs are one of those things. There has been a lot of misinformation about drugs, but it is true that certain drugs do affect sexual powers. The one that is most at fault is alcohol.

I know a lot of you men think that drinking makes you more

sexy. If you think that, you're wrong, because alcohol does exactly the opposite—it cuts you down sexually. Take the loss of potency caused by drinking and add a little fear, and you could escalate right into full-scale impotence. Let me show you how that could happen.

Here is one area where women come off better. Alcohol might have a specific effect on the ability of a man to have an erection, but it doesn't have any effect on the sexual vigor of a woman—unless, of course, she drinks herself into a stupor. In fact, a moderate amount of alcohol will increase a woman's sexual vigor.

Whereas *moderate* drinking releases inhibitions, it doesn't take long before alcohol starts to cause sexual dysfunction. That's true for both men and women, but it happens in different ways. If a man is a heavy drinker—that is, a full-fledged alcoholic—he's almost certain to be impotent. That's because alcohol will destroy the nerves that make it possible to have an erection. As I said, it works differently for a woman. Even though too much alcohol (the exact amount obviously varies from person to person) will stop her from lubricating, she can still do that artificially. She just won't want to, because after a certain point, alcohol decreases desire in everyone. So the alcohol, beyond moderation, actually stops the most important sexual function for both men and women. The difference is, the woman can perform in spite of that, and the man cannot.

Narcotics in general, especially the hard narcotics like heroin, morphine and cocaine, in excess generally depress the desire to have sex and the ability to perform.

However, the drugs you are more likely to be concerned with aren't the so-called "hard" drugs, but the drugs that are commonly used for sedatives or tranquilizers. The newspapers have been full of the ill effects of these drugs. Now while I agree that prolonged use of certain sedatives such as barbiturates can become addictive and that tranquilizers used over a long period of time can depress sexual activity, the whole problem has been over-emphasized, in my opinion.

For example, the drugs used for high blood pressure are notorious for depressing the sex drive. Some depress it by blocking impulses from the brain, and others depress it by working directly on the sex organs. Some of them can keep a man from having an erection, and some of them can make ejaculation difficult.

But . . . and it's a big "but"—recently, many authorities have agreed that those dangers have been exaggerated. While those drugs do have some effect on sexual performance, the effect is not as great as the newspapers and popular magazines would have us believe.

Anti-depressant drugs have a bad name as far as sexual potency is concerned. In fact, they are generally blamed for causing impotence. Well, they might also be victims of bad press, because several recent articles in professional journals have given cases where the drug has *increased* the sexual vigor of the person taking it by relieving the depression.

Now what about specific diseases? Well, the disease most often associated with impotence is diabetes. In fact, impotence is often one of the very first symptoms of diabetes. Does diabetes cause total impotence? Yes, sometimes it does. However, in most cases, the impotence will only be partial. By the way, "partial" impotence isn't the same kind of thing as being "a little bit" pregnant. What I mean by partial is that sometimes you can do it, and sometimes you can't. Total impotence means you always can't.

Very often, if the diabetes is brought under control, the improved general health of the person will bring back any sexual ability that was lost because of the disease.

You've got to realize, though, that everything depends on the length of time a man has been impotent. For example, take a man who has had diabetes for thirty or forty years and has been impotent for the last fifteen or twenty. I'm afraid the possibility he can be cured is very slim.

On the other hand, if the diabetes happens later in life, that's usually a much milder form of the disease, and the outlook is pretty good.

The effect of diabetes on a woman is not the same. She may lose some sensation in the genital area, but as long as she has some libido, she can perform. And with the libido can even reach orgasm.

The second most common organic cause of impotence is blood vessel disease, if it decreases the blood supply to the genital organs. I'm talking about such diseases as arteriosclerosis, or thickening of the arteries, and aneurysm, which is a thinning out and ballooning of the walls of a blood vessel. The thickening of the blood vessels restricts the flow of blood that helps make the genital organs and the lower extremities function. It's not fatal, but it can cause impotence and, for example, loss of function of the legs. The aneurysm is more dangerous. If the balloon bursts, it will be fatal. However, if those conditions are caught early enough, they can be easily corrected with surgery.

The last couple of things I've talked about have obviously been directed at men, but here's something that both men and women might find themselves having to deal with. I'm talking about the person who has had a stroke.

If you've had a stroke, you might still be able to function sexually in some way. A stroke is more likely to have a psychological effect on you than a physical one. It can be a tremendous blow to your ego to feel that you can't function as a whole person. That's when a sympathetic and understanding mate or sexual partner is a real necessity.

Many stroke victims still have the potential for functioning sexually. If that's true of you, then you can be taught—as part of the process of rehabilitation—new ways of positioning yourself so you can indulge in sexual relationships. The activity could be intercourse, or it could be manual or oral sex. But the important thing is to realize that you are still desirable, still wanted—and, best of all, can still function.

You may be wondering how sexual activity is possible if you are confined to a wheelchair. Maybe you've had the experience of being aroused and wanting to do something, but by the time your partner helps you out of the wheelchair and into bed, the desire is gone and you can't get it back. Sure, that's a problem—but only if you insist on having sex in bed. What's wrong with doing something right there in the wheelchair? There are several ways it can be done. A woman can easily sit on the man, facing away from him so he can insert his penis, or she can satisfy him with her mouth or with her hands. The man can satisfy a woman in a wheelchair either orally or manually, too. Of course, moving a woman to the bed isn't as much of a problem because she has no erection to lose.

The important thing is to keep it spontaneous. Find the easiest and quickest way to do it that is right for both of you.

Maybe you've had a heart attack and you have been wondering, "What is this going to do to my sex life? Am I going to be able to function?" And even if you haven't had a heart attack, you're probably at the age when you're starting to wonder what is going to happen to you if you did have one. Those are important questions, and they deserve answers.

To my mind, one of the greatest faults of medicine in the past was that so many physicians were reluctant to instruct their heart-attack patients about sex. If you went to one of those doctors, you got plenty of advice on diet, on exercise, on activity in general, but not one word about the subject that was uppermost in your mind— "When can I have sex again?" or even, "Can I ever have sex again?" In that part of the treatment, far, far too many physicians failed. Today, however, most physicians are bombarded with advice about the treatment of sexual dysfunctions. They are more aware of the problems and are able to give their patients good, solid advice.

Of course, if you've had a heart attack, I'm not going to start you out right away on a regimen of hectic activity and vigorous sex. That's swinging the pendulum way too far the other way. You need a period of time to recover and repair the damage that was done to the heart. That usually takes somewhere in the neighborhood of six weeks. Oh, it might take a few weeks longer in some cases, but sometimes it takes even less time.

How would I know when the time is right for you to resume sexual activity after a heart attack? Let me assure you, it's not by guesswork. There are definite standards I can apply. For instance, it's a known fact that in normal intercourse the pulse rate will triple and the blood pressure will rise as much as 30 or 40 millimeters of mercury, which is a pretty sharp rise. The rate of breathing will pick up considerably, too.

It's also a fact that when a person gets aroused emotionally or is in some kind of stress situation where tempers flare, the very same thing happens. The blood pressure goes up, the pulse gets faster, and the breathing gets heavy. Nobody gets too excited about that, do they? Well, if you can tolerate those bursts of emotion or temper without stress, you can tolerate intercourse without stress.

If you can manage to walk briskly around the block without getting short of breath or getting a pain in your chest, or if you can manage to walk up—not run up—two flights of stairs without severe shortness of breath or chest pains, then intercourse is not going to hurt you.

Once you've been given the okay to have intercourse again after a heart attack, there are some things you can do to take the strain out of it. For example, it's a good idea to let the well partner be on top, because the bottom position is by far the least strenuous. But whatever position is chosen, it should be one that allows the well partner to do all the "work," and allows you to take it as easy as possible.

For people who experience chest pain from emotional excitement, I don't hesitate to recommend putting a nitroglycerin tablet under the tongue to relieve the pain. If you have that problem and you know there is likely to be pain, take the pill before you have intercourse.

Heart attacks are scary things. You can't get around that. You probably know people who have died from them. But you probably also know people who have had heart attacks and recovered from them. The thing to remember is that it may not be as bad as you fear it is. As with many other things, the fear is often worse than the reality. If you are still skeptical about what a person who has had a heart attack can do, let me tell you about Dr. Terence Kavanagh. Dr. Kavanagh is medical director of the Toronto Rehabilitation Center. He started putting his patients on endurance exercise programs. Within a few years of starting his project, he took seven of his patients to compete in the Boston Marathon. Several of those patients had had two heart attacks. All seven of those patients ran in *and finished* the 26-mile, 385-yard race, and they were in good condition when they crossed the finish line.

Now I don't care where you look or what fantastic legends you dig up, you are never going to find a sexual act that is as exhausting as running more than twenty-six miles!

* * *

What about diseases like arthritis, chronic lung disease, spastic conditions—do they affect sexual functioning? Not directly. However, they may make the kind of moving around you do with sexual activity painful. I'd recommend taking something for the pain beforehand so you are able to relax a little more. Most pain pills—unless they are narcotic—won't dull sexual potency in any way. If you have chronic problems with breathing, the effort of sex can produce an intense shortness of breath. You can use an inhalator just before intercourse—or even during intercourse, if necessary. Stopping in the middle might be distracting at first, but you'll soon get used to doing it and not be bothered at all. I would suggest positioning yourself so you make the least possible effort.

As with most other things, the worst problem is the fear of not being able to function. If you are suffering from any of those conditions and are having trouble sexually, just be patient. I have patients with all those conditions—and they are managing to enjoy sex. They know they don't have to worry about something dreadful happening to them. They aren't about to die from the exertions of sexual activity. And that's something you should know, too.

Chapter 10:
WHAT IF YOU'VE HAD AN OPERATION?

There was a time when surgery for an older person carried a great deal of risk, and doctors were reluctant to do operations on them. Today this is no longer a problem in most cases. Because of the tremendous advances that have been made in anesthesia and other surgical areas, operations are done routinely on patients of any age—into the nineties, if necessary.

Surgery is a fact of life for an older person. The older you get, the more likely you are to need an operation of some kind. What I'm trying to tell you is you shouldn't be afraid of it just because you are older. Surprisingly enough, we have found that some older men and women recover from surgery faster than young people do. It depends on your attitude. If you are vigorous and love life and want to get well, then you've got a good chance of getting well with the ease and speed of a younger person.

Boy, I remember old Sam. He was a case! Sam was seventy-six years old, and I operated on him for a bad case of hemorrhoids. This was some years ago, when operating conditions weren't as good as they are now. Well, that vigorous seventy-six-year-old made the most rapid recovery I have ever seen after rectal surgery. It seemed like they hardly had him back from the recovery room before he was grabbing at the nurses. He was so spry they used to like to take him around to other rooms to show him off as a good example—especially to rooms where younger men were moaning and groaning about similar operations they had just been through. Sam was ninety-six this year, and still enjoying life.

Even if you know surgery is not filled with the dangers for you that it once was, I'm sure you've heard from well-meaning friends that if you have to go in for an operation, you can kiss sex good-bye. Is that true? What effect will surgery have on your sex life? Well, that's exactly what I want to talk about now.

Most of the general surgery you are likely to encounter will have little or no effect on your sexual potential. By general surgery I mean things like taking out a gall bladder, intestinal obstructions, removing an appendix. They have no effect on your sexuality at all, except for the inconvenience and the period of recovery. You'll be pretty much the same as you were before the surgery. So if you were active before the operation, you will probably be sexually active afterward.

There are some surgical problems that might cause some sexual dysfunction in the male. The most common one in the age range I'm talking about is the prostate. Any man who is over fifty is likely to have some problems with his prostate. The kind of problem will range from very simple to highly complex and serious. The treatment, of course, will vary with the severity of the problem.

Most men who have prostatic surgery are operated on for benign disease of the prostate, which simply means there is no cancer. What's more, out of the four approaches to prostatic surgery, three of them should have little or no effect on your sexual potential. Let's look at each of the different kinds in more detail.

On the simplest level, there's the natural enlargement that all men experience as a normal part of aging, with no malignancy present. Now even though there is no cancer, the enlargement is going to interfere with the normal flow of urine from the bladder. The operation to correct this problem is simple—it just involves cutting off the part of the prostate that is causing the block. The easiest way to do that is to insert an electrical instrument through the penis, which simply shaves off those pieces of the prostate that are encroaching on the urethral canal, so you can urinate freely.

Another method of approaching the benign prostate is through the abdomen. The usual reason for it is an increase in size. The third method is by making an incision in the perineum, which is the area between the scrotum and the anus. This last one is an easy approach to the prostate, but it's also an area where the risk of damage to nerves is higher. The way things break down, 95 percent of the men who have the first kind of operation will remain potent, 90 percent of those who have the abdominal operation, and about 50 percent of those who undergo the perineal approach retain the same potency they had before the operation.

The fourth kind of prostate operation is the most drastic. That is the one which involves cancer. In such a case the surgeon must remove as much of the cancerous tissue as possible, which means taking all of the prostate, the coverings around the prostate, and severing all the nerves and vessels that approach the prostate gland. The potential for any potency remaining is about 10 percent. That's not really a bad percentage, considering you're dealing with such a radical operation.

How can you tell if you have prostate trouble? The most important sign of an enlarged prostate is that you start urinating more frequently, particularly at night. If you're getting up once a night to urinate, it's not anything to worry about. Even twice a night is no cause for alarm. But if you find you have to get up three or four times a night, that's when it's time to do some checking. Another sign of trouble is the inability to hold off urinating. When you've gotta go, you've gotta go right now. You can't hold on to it in an emergency like you used to be able to. If you don't go, you find yourself dribbling before you get to the bathroom.

There is also a difference in the way you urinate when you have prostate trouble. The stream is not as forceful as it used to be. It takes longer to get started, and it's not as easy to finish—there is a tendency to dribble.

One of the results of the operation that will seem strange and will take some getting used to is a change in the way you ejaculate. What will happen is you will ejaculate backwards, into the bladder. You might be a little startled to feel all the sensations you are used to with ejaculation, but nothing comes out. Believe me, it is not harmful in any way, and it won't take you long to get used to it.

Many of you have had to deal with another kind of surgical problem—the colostomy or the ileostomy. Both operations are simply a permanent opening on the abdomen for the release of the bowel content. Colostomy is the more common for older people. While those operations themselves won't cause impotence or other sexual problems directly, they can easily do so indirectly. The feeling of being unclean, of being unacceptable to one's mate, can be enough to cause a serious sexual dysfunction.

Anyone who has had the operation needs the love, patience, and understanding of an interested and interesting partner. The partner must be able to accept the disability without showing signs of aversion or distaste. On the other hand, the person who has had the operation must show some patience and understanding, too. No matter how much the partner cares, the fact of the operation is an emotional shock. It's important to keep that in mind in case the partner doesn't always react perfectly at first.

Possibly the worst thing about a colostomy is not knowing what to expect. A man who has been told he must have the operation might have a fantasy about the future that goes something like this: "I just had a colostomy, and I don't want to touch my wife because I'm afraid she's going to draw back and not want to touch me. She's going to be disgusted. It's making me depressed, it's cutting my appetite off, and I'm losing interest in sex. I don't want that to happen."

Or if a man's wife is to be the patient, the fantasy might go this way: "My wife just had a colostomy, and I'm bringing her home from the hospital tomorrow. We had a pretty good time with sex before, and sooner or later I'm going to want to get back to that. But I've noticed a difference in her attitude toward me when I visit her in the hospital. She seems to be holding back, like she's afraid of me. I think she's wondering what it's going to be like when we get home. I don't know how I can reassure her that I'm still interested and her operation isn't going to bother me. Well, even if it does at first, I'm willing to work hard to get over it. How do I keep from turning her off if I forget and make a face or wince when I see her?"

Those are both frightening possibilities, but there's an important reality they don't take into account. If you were having a simpler operation, you would go to the hospital, have the surgery, and after recovery you'd be released. But a colostomy is far more complex, and the danger of psychological harm is too great for that kind of treatment. With a colostomy, you're not only given a period of recovery from the physical effects of the surgery, you're also given intensive counseling and help with the emotional and psychological problems you will encounter. You will be visited by members of the local cancer society and the local colostomy club. You'll be taught how to take care of your colostomy, and how to keep it clean. Your spouse will also be visited and counseled, and there will even be sessions for the two of you together. Intensive counseling and maybe even therapy might be needed, but the help is there. You will not be left to fend for yourself as best you can.

The apparatus itself is a small plastic bag that flattens out. It isn't bulky, and it doesn't show through clothing. It's not going to get in the way of sexual activity. If the idea of the bag being visible during sex bothers you, just cover it up. The opening is usually about the level of the belly button, so it's easy for a man to hide it with a T-shirt or a nightshirt. A woman can do the same with a nightgown.

Dealing with a colostomy as a married person is one thing. Your spouse will have been in on the problem since the beginning and will have learned to adjust right along with you. But suppose you're single—a widower, let's say—and you meet a woman who is attractive to you. You date for a while, and it becomes apparent the relationship is about to bloom into something more physical. Sooner or later, she is going to have to find out about your colostomy. How do you handle it? Obviously, you have to tell her about it. It would be terribly unfair to her if you just waited and let her discover it herself. Her reaction to that kind of surprise is not likely to be a balm to your ego. You will probably undo a lot of the adjustment you have made about your condition.

Be completely honest with her. Tell her all the things you were told about the operation, and how long you've had it. Assure her you are confiding in her because you know you have complete control of the problem and you don't want her to be surprised. Be careful when you tell her, to approach the subject in such a way that she can gracefully back out of the relationship if she wants to. Not everyone is going to be able to handle this kind of situation. So don't push. Someone who hesitates at first might have a change of mind later.

If you have had a colostomy or ileostomy, keep in mind that you are not alone. Many, many others have dealt with the problem in the past and will continue to do so. There are colostomy and ileostomy clubs throughout the country, made up of people who have lived for years with these operations and have adjusted to them. They have learned to live happily, have normal intercourse and normal relationships, and it doesn't make any difference in their married lives.

A very common operation for women, and one which has its own extensive mythology, is the hysterectomy. The biggest myth is that once you've had a hysterectomy, you can forget about sexual feeling for the rest of your life. Women today are much more knowledgeable about such things than they used to be, but it still astonishes me to find out how many still believe that myth. As a matter of fact, the contrary is usually true. When a younger woman has a hysterectomy, she can absolutely stop worrying about a possible unwanted pregnancy. Being relieved of that anxiety is often all that's needed to make her more vigorous sexually.

That last isn't really important for our purposes, because we're dealing with older women here. However, the myth I just mentioned is just as strong for older women as it is for anyone else. There are women who are absolutely convinced that a hysterectomy—even after menopause—will rob them of their womanhood. That's totally ridiculous, because the uterus and the ovaries have outlived their usefulness by that time. Nature reduces those organs in size as the years go on, so a woman in her seventies or eighties has a uterus no more than the size of your thumb, a little nubbin of tissue that has shrunk because it is no longer useful. It's really a natural hysterectomy. By that time the ovaries are so tiny they can hardly be found.

Women aren't the only ones to cling to this myth. Many a husband still believes that if his wife has a hysterectomy, she is going to be lost to him as a sex partner. That notion is as ridiculous as anything else. The clitoris has the same sensory nerve endings as it did before, and we know that is the focal point of sexual excitement in a woman. The vagina is still there and all the nerves in the outer part are intact, so no sensation is going to be lost there, either. Nothing is disturbed. Lubrication is as fast and efficient as it ever was. There is no loss of muscle control.

Maybe you're still doubtful. Maybe you know someone who put on weight and stopped looking attractive after a hysterectomy. If that happened to her, it happened because she wanted it to—not because of the operation. She was using the hysterectomy as an excuse to let herself go. I can show you any number of women who have had hysterectomies and are as good-looking as they ever were. They have the same joy in life as they always had.

You know, if I walked down the street—any street, anywhere—and tried to pick out twenty women who had had a hysterectomy, I couldn't do it. I couldn't pick out one. The only way I can tell if a woman has had a hysterectomy is to put her on the examining table and manually examine her uterus. It doesn't show. And no man can tell by having intercourse with a woman if she has had the operation, either.

One last thing. Very often the muscles of the vagina are slack and stretched out of shape in an older woman. It's a simple matter for the surgeon to tighten those muscles up and make you like you were when you were first married. So you see, the operation can also improve your sex life.

Another common operation for women and one with

perhaps more serious emotional overtones is the mastectomy. When a woman has had a breast removed, she has really not had anything done to destroy her sexual vigor or her sexual feelings in any way. But what has happened to her is that something has been done to her mentally. It's no secret that having a breast removed can destroy a woman's image of herself as a woman. It's a lot trickier psychologically than a hysterectomy, because she can see what's missing. Unfortunately, the culture we live in has tended to almost worship a woman's breasts as a symbol of sexuality and beauty. She not only has to deal with the fact that she can tell it's missing, but her husband or sexual partner can, too.

A mastectomy brings with it a second problem. After all, why does a woman have a breast removed? The breast is removed because of cancer. So she not only has to deal with the problem of not feeling like a whole woman, she has to worry about whether or not all the cancer was gotten out of her. Will she survive?

This is another time when much love, patience, and understanding are needed. If you've had a mastectomy, you need a husband or a partner who is going to be able to let you know that the loss of a breast has not made you any less attractive or any less desirable to him and he still loves you as much as ever and enjoys you as much as ever.

Those things work both ways, you know. So it's up to you to let him know you accept this love from him without reservation, and to let him know you feel very much a woman.

In many cases, plastic surgery is possible, so an artificial breast can be constructed with a silicone implant and it will look and feel like the real thing. That's much easier to do if only the breast itself has been removed. But even if the surrounding tissue has been removed, such an implant is still possible. You're likely to have to wait for some time, though, until the doctor is sure all the cancer has been removed.

All the kinds of counseling I have mentioned for people who have had colostomies and ileostomies are available for women who have had mastectomies. And there are also special clubs for people who have had the operation. Be assured that you are not going to be alone. You will always be able to find someone who has been there, too, and who understands your special needs.

The right kind of attitude and a refusal to give in to groundless fears about yourself can do a great deal to keep you sexually alive and vital.

Chapter 11:
HAVING (AND BEING) AN INTERESTING AND INTERESTED PARTNER

In order to have a satisfying sex life, you need an interesting and interested partner. That's true no matter what your age, but it's especially true as you get older. I've mentioned this before—more than once, in fact—but I haven't said enough about what I mean by an "interesting and interested" partner. Let's take care of that right now.

Do I mean a movie star, famous author, adventurer, astronaut or other kind of celebrity? Not at all. A person can be interesting without being world famous. As a matter of fact, a person can be world famous without being interesting.

Interesting means there's an aura of aliveness about you. You talk about things you and your partner are interested in—that could be your work, your hobby, your views on the news of the day. Or maybe you talk about a book you have just finished, and you find your views are different enough that you and your partner could spend several hours discussing it. It could mean discussing your likes and dislikes about a movie you saw together.

You can be interesting in the way you carry yourself, the way you take care of your appearance. If you look as if you care, people are going to find you interesting. Being interesting is mostly a matter of how you feel about yourself. If you feel good about yourself and like yourself and think you are good company, chances are your partner is going to think so, too.

When I was dating after my wife died, I had definite ideas about what I wanted my companion to be like. I wanted her to be attractive and to care about how she looked. I wanted her to be able to hold up her end of the conversation and be a good listener, too. I wanted her to be someone I felt good about introducing to my friends and family. I also wanted her to have enough regard for herself to make the same kinds of demands on me. In other words, I didn't want an emotional doormat.

You know, it's almost impossible for two people to get together in the first place if they aren't interested in each other. Very often that interest is generated by a shared activity. Maybe you were both tennis players or swimmers. You met at the courts or in the pool, and that's what brought you together. Then as your relationship developed, you found other things that were interesting.

Or it might work the other way. You might have gotten together in the first place because of your differences. A couple might come together at a party. She finds out he is an accomplished amateur musician, and he discovers she is an excellent photographer. The relationship takes hold because they each find it interesting to share and discover new ideas and experiences.

The point is that you are receptive to the other person's interests, even though they might not be yours. No two people can have the same interests all the time. Very few people maintain common interests all through their lives.

An important point to remember is that whatever triggered the original interest will continue to be an important part of the relationship. Very often, when that starts to slip, the relationship starts to slip.

Take a patient of mine, for example. He and his wife first met because he was interested in music. He played the guitar, even wrote a lot of his own songs. He had an income from various trusts and investments, so he didn't have to work. He kept himself busy with athletics. He worked out, he jogged, he swam, he played tennis. Then he began to lose interest in his

Having an Interesting and Interested Partner 133

music. He stopped writing songs; he stopped getting together with other musicians; and then his guitar started collecting dust. His wife got tired of seeing the thing lying around the house, so she put it in its case and stuck it away in a closet. He never bothered to ask her where it was.

The next thing to go was the exercise. He began to spend more and more time sitting around the house daydreaming. It began to irritate his wife, having him underfoot all the time. That was the way she described it to me, which was funny, because he wasn't around the house any more than he had been before. The difference was that he was no longer interesting to her. Their sexual activity dropped to zero.

Whenever there is a falling-off of interest in another person, it can usually be traced back to one specific incident. So the first thing I'd like you to ask yourself is, when did it happen? Can you think of one specific thing that suddenly made you change the way you felt about your partner? Can you pinpoint anything that might have been the start of your problem? What was it that made you believe you were sexually dysfunctional, that you couldn't perform?

Being an interesting partner is something that works both ways, you know. If your partner is not interesting to you, the chances are that you are not very interesting to your partner, either. In fact, you can take that one step further and say if you aren't very interesting to yourself, you aren't going to be very interesting to your partner.

Being interested in yourself is absolutely essential to being healthy emotionally. Once you lose that vital interest in yourself, things can start to go to hell pretty rapidly. The patient I just talked about is a good example of that. Then when you start to slip, the whole thing can get to be kind of a vicious circle. One person in a relationship lets down, and the other one thinks, "Oh, what's the use? Why should I bother?"

Take a good look at yourself. What have you done with yourself lately? Do you still try to keep yourself attractive? Do you still take care of yourself and the way you look? Do you dress as carefully as you did when you were younger? Have you tried to stay trim and healthy looking or have you let your figure go to pot?

Are you as careful about bodily cleanliness as you once

were? Do you bathe regularly, brush your teeth often, keep your hair looking neat and clean? You men out there—do you still shave every day or have you started to get careless about that?

What about your clothing? Do you try to look sharp and take care of your clothes, or do you just throw on the first thing you see when you get dressed in the morning—no matter if it's dirty, torn, or wrinkled?

People can't tell what's on your mind. They don't know what you're thinking about yourself. What you've got to do is advertise. You tell them about yourself by what you wear, how neat you are, how you take care of yourself in general. And don't forget your partner. Being able to be proud of you is an important thing. How do you think he or she feels, seeing the loss of the interest your friends used to have in you?

A man who isn't interested anymore in how he looks will soon lose interest in his surroundings. Take a man who used to be very neat about his person, and therefore was very neat about his belongings. He took care of his clothes; he hung things up; he put books and magazines away when he was finished reading them. He didn't leave things cluttering up the house. Then he starts getting careless about his appearance, and before long everything else starts slipping, too. If he used to help his wife around the house, he stops doing that and lets her do everything.

The same kind of thing happens with a woman. She loses interest in keeping up the house, so instead of coming home to a cheerful, neat house, she comes into something that is well on its way to becoming a dump.

But that's not all there is to it. What do you do to make yourself interesting to talk to and to listen to? Do you still try to keep up with what's going on in the world, or do you find that the only time your conversation changes is when the weather changes? Have you tried to keep up your hobbies or find new ones? Are you taking advantage of your leisure time to find special things to do for fun, or are you just sitting and watching your life trickle away?

You would probably be astonished to know how many sexual problems are caused by the simple fact that a couple has gotten into a rut in everyday living. After work they eat dinner and then they sit in front of the television set until it is time to go to bed. The only way they can tell one day from another is that the TV programs are different. They haven't been out to a movie or to the theatre together since—who knows when. Once in a while they go to somebody's house to play cards or for a party.

If a couple like that had a satisfying sexual relationship, I would be astonished to hear about it. They aren't really interested in life, much less in each other. And yet when such couples come to me for counseling—and they do—all too often the man will tell me his wife is frigid!

What do I tell a man like that? Well, the first thing I say to him is, if you treated your wife that way when you were courting her, you wouldn't have gotten to first base!

It's not that people aren't able to be interesting to each other, you know. When people are just dating, and even in the courtship phase of the relationship, they break their necks to be attractive and interesting to each other.

So I will tell a man who complains about having a frigid wife, if you treated her like you did before you were even interested in marrying her and you were on the make for her, you wouldn't have a frigid wife. She certainly wasn't frigid the first year or two you were married. Now suddenly she is.

Just think back to when you were dating. Did you try to take her to bed without any preliminaries? Of course you didn't! You took her to a show, you took her to dinner, you took her to a bar for a couple of drinks, you went dancing—in short, you did things with her and got interested in things with her.

That's what you've got to start doing now. Think about it. It worked back then, didn't it? What makes you think it wouldn't work now? Yes, that will mean some effort, but you don't get the results without the effort. And you wouldn't be reading this book if you didn't want the results.

That's one kind of rut a couple can fall into, but it's not the only one. Maybe the problem is simply that there is not enough variety in your sex life. Sex can get boring if it's the same old thing all the time. The solution to that problem could be as easy as trying different positions for intercourse. That's perfectly all right for you to do, you know. As long as you and your partner find a position comfortable and enjoyable, there's nothing wrong with it. Just be sure you *both* enjoy it and find it comfortable.

Another way to put some variety into your relationship is for you women to occasionally take over initiating sexual contact. Oh, I know, that's not an easy thing to think about. Most older women were brought up in an atmosphere that discouraged the very idea of a woman making the first move. Starting up a sexual encounter has always been thought to be the man's job. Or maybe you're afraid to try it because you think you might turn your man off with aggressive behavior.

Yes, that could happen. You could be so aggressive that you might scare your man away. But frankly, if you've got any common sense at all, I don't think there's much danger of that happening. You don't have to come on strong. In fact, you don't have to come on much at all. You know, I'm not suggesting you grab your guy and say, "Okay, fella, how about a roll in the hay?"

What am I suggesting then? Well, for example, why don't you get out an especially seductive perfume your husband has commented on—it's better if you have one you haven't used for a while. Put it on, and the next thing you know he's going to start getting ideas. He's going to say to himself, "I wonder why she's putting on that perfume? I bet she's interested." That's all there is to it. You do that, and you have actually made the first move. Now it's up to him.

There are other things you can do that are just as subtle. For example, many of the women I counsel are shy about appearing nude in front of their husbands, and they don't like to undress in front of them. You can use that kind of shyness very effectively to start a sexual contact—and even if you aren't shy at all, it's still going to work.

There is nothing more stimulating to a man than to see a woman partially undressed, or in the process of undressing. That's why I advise dressing in the dressing room with the door partially open, and making sure that while you appear to be doing it in private, he can see everything that is going on.

If you usually go to bed with a heavy nightgown, trade it for a flimsy one from time to time. If you really are shy—and even if you are not—put a robe on, but leave it open at the front. Then walk in front of him in such a way that he can't help but see through that thing.

You may be used to making love in the dark. Well, you might try subtly turning on a nightlight and then "forgetting" to turn it off when you get into bed.

Do you always go to bed with curlers in your hair? One night, leave the curlers off. You always go to bed with grease on your face? Don't grease it—do that afterward.

Almost anything you do like that is going to have some effect. Your partner isn't going to need to have a building fall on his head to realize those things are happening for a reason. It doesn't take much to give a man the idea that you are interested. You don't have to come right out and say, "Let's make love." All you have to do is give the guy the idea—and if he's on the ball, he'll pick up on it.

But what if he doesn't pick up on it? What if he misses the signals completely? In that case, you can either try something a little bolder, or you can just let it go—and you haven't lost face or been embarrassed.

Anytime you women do take the lead, remember one thing—*never* force the issue. That's especially true if your man has some trouble getting or maintaining an erection. Be content to just lie there and be pleasant, and at no time give him the notion that you expect him to perform. You can tell him, "Honey, it feels good just to lie next to you and hold you." Let him know you like to be held, that it's comfortable for you and you get a lot of pleasure from it.

You can tell him how you would like to be fondled, or even guide his hand to the places you want to be caressed. Just don't make him think any of this is an indication you want him to perform. If he responds to what is happening, then he'll take over from there. But if he doesn't respond, let him know that you're content with what he's doing.

You might wonder why I'm talking about the idea of sexual performance right now. One of the problems I have to deal with a lot in my own practice is the man who avoids starting any kind of sexual activity with his wife. It sounds like the same problem women have, doesn't it? Well, the reason for it is a little different. With women, the reason is usually upbringing or shyness. With men, it's fear. Fear of starting something he may not be able to finish.

There is a man I'm treating right now who finally admitted to that problem. At first, he was able to have an erection, but he couldn't maintain it. Then it got to the point where he began to have difficulty in getting an erection at all. His way of dealing with the problem was to avoid sex as much as possible. Fortunately, his wife's way of dealing with it was to seek help. The man finally admitted to me that he really wanted to fondle his wife, caress her, and be affectionate with her—but he was afraid that every time he tried it she would think he was going to perform. The fear of failure put so much pressure on him that he often did fail, which eroded his ego and his ability even more. When he came to me, he told me that in the preceding year he had made only two attempts.

The first thing I told him—told the two of them, in fact—was *don't perform.* Even if you get your first erection in months, don't attempt intercourse. When *can* you attempt intercourse? That varies from person to person. My rule of thumb is, when you've had enough erections from the stimulation of caressing and being caressed to be reassured that it isn't just a freak occurrence, then you can try intercourse.

The reason for that, of course, was to take the onus of performance away from the man entirely. Telling him in the presence of his wife is additional reassurance for him that she is not going to expect performance from him. It is going to take time to correct his problem, but at least he and his wife can share cuddling and affection without fear. Hopefully, the situation will reverse itself, and they will again be able to enjoy a full sexual relationship together.

One of the commonest causes of loss of interest by one partner is the sickness of the other partner. Illness is not a pleasant thing under any circumstances. Even so, we find it fairly easy to be sympathetic and helpful and loving to the one who is sick—up to a point. There are many people who continue to baby themselves after an illness. They moan and they groan, and they use the sickness as an excuse to be waited

Having an Interesting and Interested Partner 139

on hand and foot and to keep from having to get back into circulation. You get tired very quickly of a chronic complainer. No matter how much you love a person, you can only bear to hear the sighs and the complaints for so long. Then it becomes a royal pain in the neck.

I have patients who have arthritis and won't make a move, no matter how many times I tell them the more mobile they are, the less likely they are to be crippled by the condition. But no, they would rather sit around and whine and wonder why nobody is particularly interested in their company anymore.

Now let's get back to being an interesting partner.

If your problem has been that you are in a rut, then do something about it! Start going out with your friends, start visiting more. Have people over to your home. Find a common hobby—or each of you find your own hobby and share your excitement and interest with each other. Let yourself be interested in the things your partner is interested in.

One of the most important things you can do together is to exercise together. Nothing can stimulate a body more than exercising. Exercise will get the circulation, lungs, and all your vital organs to function better than ever. Exercise will not only help your sex life, it will also improve every other aspect of your health and well-being.

Always consult your doctor before you start any kind of regular exercise—and that includes walking. If you have doubts about your capacity or you've had any kind of heart problem, ask your doctor about an exercise tolerance test. That will give you an accurate indication of the capacity of your heart for exercise and the limits to which it can be pushed. You'll know just what you can and cannot do.

There are several good exercises you can do together that are good for your general physical condition and are good for keeping your weight down. The simplest and easiest of them all is walking. Another advantage of walking is you don't need any special equipment for it. So get in the habit of walking a mile or two every day. Now I don't mean "window-shopping" type walking. I mean walking where you move out briskly for a mile or two.

A word of warning about walking, which also applies to

other kinds of exercise. Start out gradually. You don't go out and walk two miles at top speed the first day. If you do that, you're just asking for trouble. Start out with a couple of blocks and build it up over a period of time. If you get short of breath or a pain in the chest, or you feel nausea, stop at once. Those are signs you are overdoing it. A good way to pace yourself is to talk as you walk. If you can carry on a conversation without strain, you're not overdoing. But if you find it hard to talk, slow down until you are comfortable. That's a technique used to train long-distance runners, and it really works!

If walking doesn't appeal to you, how about swimming or bicycling? What about tennis, or jogging, or skipping rope? Fine—if your doctor says okay. Golf is a good exercise, but you have to walk for it to do you any good. The average course is between four and five miles long. If you forego the golf cart and walk briskly between shots, you're going to get plenty of exercise. Another thing—it keeps you out of doors for four or five hours.

Another word of caution about exercise—it must be regular. If you're going to walk, walk daily. If you bicycle, do it at least three or four times a week, and the same for swimming. But if you only swim one day a week, then walk the other days. Whatever you do, don't limit your exercise to weekends or your one or two days off, because that kind of irregular strain is dangerous to your body.

I read something another doctor wrote once which has really stuck in my mind— "If you want to know when you will die, be a weekend athlete. You'll die on a weekend."

Learning to relax is also important, and more and more ways of doing that are becoming available. I'm talking about things like meditation and yoga, for example. There's nothing more inviting or more pleasant in a sexual relationship than a completely relaxed person whose whole mind and body are involved in the fun and pleasure of the sexual experience— without the mind being way off somewhere thinking of a million other things.

A very simple way of relaxing—which I use myself—is to sit in a comfortable chair or lie down and very slowly breathe in and out and say to yourself each time you breathe in and out,

"I'm feeling more and more relaxed." You'll gradually feel yourself go limp. Or you can concentrate on making one part of your body at a time relax: "I'm relaxing my right foot. I'm relaxing my right leg. I'm relaxing my left foot. I'm relaxing my left leg. I'm relaxing my right thigh," and so forth. Pretty soon you'll feel yourself become very limp and rested. After you get good at those techniques, doing one for five or ten minutes can make you feel like you've had a good night's sleep. You feel relaxed and refreshed. These kinds of exercise also teach us to concentrate on what we're doing at the moment, prevent our being easily distracted, help us to "go with" what we're doing. Thus they help us in our sexual experiences.

Now let's talk a little about what I mean when I say you must have an "interested" partner. A lot more is known these days about what makes people tick sexually. One of the things we know is that sexual dysfunction is never a one-person problem. It is always a two-person problem. A man who is sexually dysfunctional is not dysfunctional all by himself, he is dysfunctional with his partner. To treat one of them without treating the other would be not only improper, it would be almost sure to fail.

What if you have a problem and your partner isn't willing to go along with counseling or therapy? Unfortunately, the answer in that case is, you can't do anything. If one partner is not interested in coming in at all, there is no way you can resolve the problem. Unfortunately, that makes treatment extremely difficult. If the person who comes in to see me is the one with the problem, I can work around the handicap of not having them both there. But if the partner is the one with the problem, then the one who comes to see me has to be, in effect, his or her own therapist. One thing I can do is show the person how to take a sexual history of the partner and help with the interpretation. A book I might recommend is one called *Making Love, How to Be Your Own Sex Therapist,* by Patricia E. Raley. However, all that is really doing it the hard way, and it will be rough going at best.

As a matter of fact, if both of them do come for counseling or therapy when they have a problem, they automatically qualify as "interested partners." I assume that if a couple comes to me for therapy, they are interested enough in themselves and their marital situation to want help. I'm also assuming the couple has no profound marital difficulties or problems between them that would get in the way of creating a good sexual union, no matter how good the therapy.

All too often, that's not the case. Sometimes during the initial interview I detect a definite animosity between the two of them that I know is going to interfere with any attempts to create sexual harmony. If that's the case, I insist they get marital counseling first. After the marital conflicts have been taken care of, then I can deal with the sexual dysfunction.

Which brings me to another important point—don't hesitate, ever, to come to your doctor with your sexual problems. Many doctors don't ask about sexual difficulties as a matter of routine when they are taking a medical history, and people are afraid to talk to their doctors about these problems—so the subject never comes up.

It's a frustrating situation, but it's easy enough to understand. People in our age group just didn't talk about sex in our youth, in our growing up period, and we don't talk about it now, except those who are highly liberated. And yet we do think about it, because in every lecture I've given I've talked to standing-room-only crowds. Afterward, there are always many, many questions asked of me. That's fine, but what has to happen is for people to go to their own doctors to get firsthand information about their own problems.

These days, the subject of sexual dysfunction is taught in the medical schools, and the professional literature and the journals are full of advice to doctors on how to deal with sexual problems. Most doctors are swamped with that kind of information. Give them a chance to use it! Even if they can't counsel you or don't feel comfortable doing so, they will be able to refer you to someone who can help.

Most important, if you need and want help, you should not wait months—or even years—before you seek it.

Chapter 12:
SPECIFIC MALE PROBLEMS

The title of this chapter says I'm going to talk to you about specific male problems. Well, I can't think of a male problem that's more specific than failure to have an erection. As a matter of fact, most of the time that's the problem that brings the patient in to see me in the first place. It's easy to understand why.

Maybe that shouldn't be such a big deal, but it is. In our society, men are conditioned to equate their sexual power with their basic manhood. Loss of sex means loss of manhood, and loss of manhood means loss of self-respect. It can destroy a person's concept of himself as a total man. The myth that your manhood is centered in your erect penis is one of the things that makes it so difficult to treat the condition, because it creates anxiety, fear, and tension.

We've talked about impotence in a general way before, but now I want to focus on just one kind—the kind we doctors like to call "functional" impotence. If that sounds like a contradiction in terms to you, it's not. "Functional" in this sense simply means the impotence is psychological in origin.

Let me give you an example of a functional disorder. If you

came to me with a headache I couldn't find a specific physical cause for, I would say it was from nervous tension and describe it as a "functional headache." If I find a heart murmur that has no specific organic cause and there is no history of previous heart disease—such as rheumatic fever, damage to a valve, or congenital deformity—I would consider that a functional murmur.

I know that talking to you by means of a book puts some limits on the kind of help I can give you and the kinds of problems I can deal with. That's why my goal in this book is to reach the many of you who can be helped sexually without long, intensive periods of therapy or direct medical attention. For that reason, I'm going to limit myself to dealing with functional impotence, although I may touch on organic problems when I mention certain diseases.

Even though the failure to have an erection is what first brings the sexual problem to my attention, the treatment always includes both partners. A sexual problem is never the problem of only one person, as I've said. It always involves two people, and therefore the therapy must be for two people. That's my procedure, and it's the procedure of most of the doctors and therapists I know. Now that's fine if you're married but what if you're single? All right, let's suppose you're a single man and you're dating somebody and sleeping with her. All of a sudden you start having sexual problems. What they are doesn't really matter at this point. You want to see somebody about the problem, but if both of you have to go, how are you going to do it?

Simple. You just bring your partner along. I never said I only treated married people. I'm sure that's true of virtually all other sex counselors as well. The basic problem a therapist would have to deal with will be the same whether you and your partner are married or not. What if you are having relations with more than one woman at a time? In that case, I would say you very likely don't have a problem.

Still, there might be good reasons why it would be difficult or even impossible for you to come in with your sexual partner if you are single. You might not have that regular a relationship, for example. Or maybe your partner simply refuses to have anything to do with going in for counseling. It's really nothing to worry about. Although it is difficult to treat just one person, the problem is one that comes up often enough for most therapists to be able to deal with it.

However, there is something I see more often than I would like to when I treat both partners. They are very likely to start hurling accusations at one another, to try and blame each other for what went wrong. That's the best sign that sexual counseling will fail without marital counseling. I can't stress this point enough—there is absolutely no room for blame in dealing with any sexual dysfunction. The only way for treatment or therapy to work is if each partner can say—and believe—"It's not your fault or my fault. Somehow between us we failed, and therefore somehow between us we've got to correct the situation." To my mind, the most important word in that statement is the word "we."

So now let's suppose you have come to see me because you have gone a while without having an erection and you're worried about it. I'm going to have to assume two things. First, that you've been examined by your doctor and he has assured you there's nothing organically wrong; and second, that your sexual partner will be reading this right along with you. You are going to need her full cooperation with the treatments I'll be suggesting.

I also want to put your mind at ease about something right at the beginning. You are *not* going to be asked to try to perform sexually. In fact, it's going to be just the opposite—I'm going to forbid you to try at all for a while. Why am I making such a big deal out of this? Because if you don't try to perform, there is no way you can fail. I want you to get the word "failure" out of your mind. I want you to be able to keep your mind on things you know you can do, not on something you fear you aren't able to do.

I've told you this in various ways before, but it's one of those things that bears repeating. The most frequent cause of functional impotence is fear—the fear of not being able to perform. Once that fear takes hold, it can set up a vicious circle that is very difficult to break.

You'll remember that there are several ways functional

impotence can begin. Illness, depression, or severe emotional shock will do it—but then, so will any other condition that produces anxiety, such as financial worries or job pressures, for example. Even if the problem is triggered by illness or depression, anxiety comes into the picture very quickly. And with the anxiety comes fear—the kind of fear that quickly kills whatever sexual desire and ability you might have. One of the most common ways of perpetuating that fear is what Masters and Johnson have called "spectatoring." What does that mean? Well, it means that you are looking at yourself from outside and evaluating what you are doing, instead of just doing it. It's as if an actor were to "watch" himself perform, instead of "being" the character. When you do that, you're not participating, because you're on the outside looking in. You're trying to will an erection or an orgasm that, after all, must happen spontaneously.

Anytime a man asks himself, "Can I still do it?" he is in trouble. It's bad enough to ask that question when you are young and you have less reason to doubt your abilities. But if you ask that question when you are older and your body has begun to slow down, the results can be really devastating.

The first thing I want you to do is forget about your genital area completely for now. What you—and your partner—are going to learn is that you have many other parts of your body which can give you pleasurable sensations. A good way to discover them is by massage.

I'm assuming that you've taken my earlier advice about learning more about yourself and your partner. So you've looked each other over carefully, your entire bodies. You're both interested in each other, so you're going to find out what parts of your bodies are sensitive to stimulation. That's what I mean by massage.

A good way to start out is to do it with your clothes on. Just go over your partner's body and stroke her all over gently and find out what she likes and what she finds stimulating. Don't touch the genital areas, though. That's very important. You'll notice I said genital *areas*. I don't mean just the primary sex organs, I mean the secondary sexual areas as well. They are the buttocks for both men and women, the nipples for men, and the breasts for women.

Then she can do the same for you, and it's up to you to let her know where you are sensitive and where it feels good to be rubbed.

By the way, the one article of clothing you should remove at this stage is shoes. The feet are a nice area to touch and have touched, but not with shoes on.

You've got to do this every day, even though in the beginning it might seem like nonsense. You may find yourself laughing at it, but pretty soon the amusement will turn into a sense of satisfaction as you begin to realize how many areas of your body can respond to stimulation. How long should you spend on it each time? The length of time doesn't really matter, as long as you are both satisfied with it and you each are massaged the same amount.

After a few days, you might want to start removing your outer clothes and do the massaging in your underwear or nightclothes. Or you can turn the session into a little striptease. Take off an article of clothing, do a little massage, take off another bit of clothing, do a little more massage, and so forth. Eventually you'll both be naked, and then you can begin the second stage of the massage. You may want to try massaging with some kind of oil. I recommend using a baby oil. You might want to add a few drops of your favorite cologne or perfume to the oil to enhance your sensory pleasure. Try the massage both with the oil and without and see which you prefer.

Of course, the ban on touching the genital areas still goes. I'll let you know when it's all right, but until then—hands off.

Now that the preliminaries are over, it's time to begin a more specific kind of massage. What you will be doing is concentrating on one particular part of the body at a time. We'll start at the bottom, with the feet. Massage her feet, and only her feet, for about twenty minutes. I can almost hear many of you saying, "What, twenty minutes massaging the feet? I'll get tired as hell." No, you won't. You'll find yourself getting a lot of pleasure from gently rubbing her that way.

Keep the massaging gentle. It should be stroking, and it

should be affectionate. Don't go at it like you're in the steam room at the gym. Try to make your partner feel it's as much of a pleasure to give the massage as to receive it. You want a little incentive to do a good job? Well, just remember—your turn is next.

After you finish with her feet, then switch off and let her do yours for the same length of time. When it's time to switch again, change the focus to another part of the body. So you start at the bottom with the feet, then do the legs and thighs, move up to the head and neck, then the trunk and the arms and shoulders. Don't forget the hands. I think you'll be surprised how good it feels to have your hands massaged.

At this point, you are not trying to get excited. You are not trying to have an erection. You might get an erection at this point, because you are getting a good deal of pleasure from touching her. If that should happen, I don't want you to do a damn thing about it. I don't care how long it's been since you've had one—leave it alone.

Do this kind of massaging several times a day, if you can, and for as long as it feels good to you. I don't care at this point if it gives you any erotic sensation. All I want is for both of you to learn what your bodies feel like to the touch. After about a week of this, more or less, you can move on to the next stage.

For this part of the massage, I want you to take a specific position. I want you to sit up with your back against the headboard and your partner sitting between your legs with her back to you. Why the fancy position? Because this time around we're going to massage the genitals. Don't get too eager, now. I want that to be the last area you touch.

All right, now, begin the massage. Go all the way around. You'll both begin to tingle, and it wouldn't surprise me if your hand is directed toward certain critical areas just a little sooner than you might expect. But don't be rushed. Keep those areas for last. Remember, gentle is the key word.

When it's your turn to have her massage you, lie on your back and have her either straddle your legs or kneel between them. That's the best position for her to have direct access to the front of your body and your genital areas. This is the time when you're likely to get an erection. And don't say, "Hey, here it is! Let's use it!" That's the one thing I don't want you to do. In fact, if you were being treated by me in person, I'd be a little upset if you came back to me and told me you tried to use it. Why? I'll tell you why. No matter how excited you are, you are almost certain to fail. At this point I'd rather not have you worry about failure.

However, if you can't resist the attempt and it works—fine, you've cured yourself. You've assured yourself it's possible to have an erection and keep it long enough to do something with it. Just don't be surprised if it fails you. That's what's most likely to happen. You have to expect it. But once again, I'd like to remind you, there is always a next time. There will be another day and another chance to try.

Now, if you've done the massages long enough to find out how many pleasant ways there are of enjoying each other, you've made a long step toward recovery. If you've seen at least the beginning of an erection, or had a full erection, you know your goal is possible.

At this point, I want you to do the massage and at the end of it try intercourse. When your partner finishes massaging you, you'll be in a good position to try it. The best way to try it is in the woman superior position. If she can put the penis into the vagina, so much the better. That seems to make it easier for the man to maintain an erection than if he tries to put it in himself. It's a good idea for her not to move until you get used to the feeling of being inside her. Many times a partially erect penis will become fully erect once it's contained in the vagina.

By the way, I don't want you to think this can all be done in a couple of evenings. You should spend a week—or at least several days—on each stage.

If you fail, what do you do? You keep trying! It might take you a while to be successful, but when you consider that your biggest fear at the beginning was that you would *never* be able to get an erection, any length of time at all is relatively short.

The important thing to remember is that if you once get to the point where you are able to have an erection, you can do it again. So don't be discouraged. The next time might be the one that works!

Getting an erection at all is one thing, but keeping the

erection once you've got it is another thing entirely. As a matter of fact, the inability to maintain an erection is the next most common sexual problem men have. If that's what's happening to you, you'll find that you don't have a lot of trouble getting an erection, but as soon as you start to use it, as soon as you try to put it in the vagina, it collapses.

Again, it's the fear of failure. It doesn't take very much to get the problem started. All it takes is for you to get an erection, penetrate the vagina, and then suddenly go soft. It could happen for any number of reasons. I don't think the reason it happens is as important as the way you react to it. If you can shrug it off and say, "It happened—so what! It'll be okay next time," and then forget about it, you're probably going to be all right.

But if you say, "What's wrong?" and the next time you get an erection you wonder if you are going to be able to keep it, you are on the way to getting a whopping big case of "fear of performance."

So I'll say the same thing I'd say if you couldn't get an erection at all—don't perform! And bear in mind that as you get older, you are simply not going to have as firm an erection as you did when you were young. But the erection you do have will be adequate to do the job.

Your partner can often be of considerable help by using the female superior position and learning how to insert a limp penis into her vagina. She can then hold the penis in by contracting her muscles.

I always caution my patients not to try to have an orgasm with a limp penis. You know, it is possible to ejaculate with a limp penis. Maybe you've even done it yourself. But if you can't maintain an erection, ejaculating with a limp penis is only going to make the problem worse. The danger is that you will get so used to doing it that way, your real goal will get lost in the shuffle. And that goal is to be able to keep an erection long enough to ejaculate with an erect penis.

You should be aware that it is not uncommon for men in the older age groups to have an erect penis and be able to penetrate, and then have it go away in the vagina. If that happens, the best thing to do is withdraw and start some kind of foreplay that will excite you until the penis becomes erect again. Just remember to withdraw if you go limp, and don't try to force yourself to ejaculate with a limp penis.

There are many mechanical devices on the market that are supposed to help a man maintain an erection, and I'm asked about them quite often. How do I feel about them? Well, some of them are useful, and others are downright dangerous. One of the dangerous ones is the ring that is put around the base of the penis to hold the congested blood in. Such a ring will keep the penis erect, but it will also cut off the circulation, and that usually does more harm than good.

A device I have on occasion recommended is the dildo—a hollowed-out artificial penis into which a man can insert his own penis. There is no sensation for the man with those things, because they have to be thick and rigid enough to penetrate.

But sometimes the fact that he's able to satisfy his partner can even excite a man to the point where he gets a good erection inside the device. And just the fact that he is doing anything at all can be enough to satisfy a man. Before surgical corrections for the problem were developed, I prescribed a dildo for a man who had become impotent from a spinal-cord injury he received in a fall. He was so delighted with the device that he wore out three of them in a matter of four years!

I'm often asked about oils and creams that are supposed to help keep an erection. There is no such thing, although people have been trying to develop one for centuries. Even such an illustrious man as Maimonides, a twelfth century rabbi, physician and philosopher, tried his hand at that kind of magic potion. Among other things, his recipe called for two pounds of live yellow ants! Needless to say, if it had worked it would still be in use today.

As a last resort, there are two surgical procedures which have been developed lately. One is the insertion of a flexible silicone sponge in the penis. The result is a constant erection, although the sponges are flexible enough now so that they can be tucked away in the shorts and don't show through the clothing.

The second operation is far more involved and expensive. The reason it costs so much more is that it pretty much duplicates the action of a normally functioning penis. A reservoir is implanted underneath the abdomen and is filled with liquid. An inflatable silicone sponge is placed in the penis, and when desired, the liquid from the reservoir is pumped to it, making the penis become erect. The pump, which is hidden in the scrotum, fills the silicone sponge with the liquid just the way blood fills the tissues in a natural erection. After intercourse, the penis can be deflated.

These operations are not something you can just ask for and receive. No surgeon will do them unless the patient has first undergone a thorough psychological evaluation.

Another male sexual problem that I encounter in my practice is premature ejaculation. Premature ejaculation is usually a problem with young men, rather than older men. The biggest problem is that if a man has been a premature ejaculator all his life, he is going to be harder to cure.

There are two methods of treating premature ejaculation which are generally used. The first is the "squeeze" technique, developed by Masters and Johnson. In the squeeze technique, the woman uses the first two fingers and the thumb. When she feels—or the man indicates—that ejaculation is about to take place, she squeezes just below the head of the penis until the urge goes away. The man is then brought to the point of ejaculation again, and the squeeze is repeated. This technique can be used with intercourse, but it is also quite effective with masturbation. If it is done with masturbation, the man can do it for himself, without the help of a partner.

The second technique—called Seaman's technique—can also be done with either manual masturbation or intercourse. Just before ejaculation, the penis is withdrawn from the vagina or the masturbation is stopped, and then the man waits until the penis begins to relax and lose its erection. At that point, the excitement process is started all over again. The process is repeated until the man learns to maintain control by himself.

One problem with both methods is that the elderly man doesn't have the two-stage ejaculatory phase of the young man, when he has the definite sensation of being about to ejaculate. With the older man, it may happen all of a sudden. So the timing has to be learned by trial and error.

Specific Male Problems

Of the techniques, I prefer the Seaman's, simply because there is less chance of injury. A woman may not know how hard to squeeze and could easily hurt the man by squeezing too hard. However, I recommend both methods in my practice, and I find they both work about equally well.

You see a lot of material in print about women who can't reach orgasm, but that's a problem men have, too. Especially older men. You may have been able to reach orgasm easily when you were younger, but now you may be having trouble. Before you start worrying that you are dysfunctional, you should keep in mind that as you get older, you have a definite reduced need to ejaculate.

The fact is, you can have a great deal of pleasure with normal sexual functioning if you stop worrying whether or not you are going to ejaculate. If you leave your body to its own devices, you will ejaculate when you need to, and you won't ejaculate when you don't need to. But if you try to force yourself to ejaculate, you are more than likely going to fail.

The first thing that's going to happen when you fail is that you are going to feel inadequate. If that happens, that's a shame, because there's no need for you to feel inadequate at all. Remember, your partner's responses are slowed by aging, too, and by not ejaculating you will be able to prolong the act enough to easily satisfy her. You're going to wind up being a terrific lover!

In fact, Masters and Johnson have said time and again that a man who ejaculates only when his body demands it, and who doesn't force it at other times, can keep his sexual vigor into his seventies, eighties—and even nineties! If you think of it that way, it doesn't seem so bad at all, does it?

Chapter 13:
SPECIFIC FEMALE PROBLEMS

What's the most common female sexual problem I see in my own practice? I'm sure it will come as no surprise to you if I tell you it is failure to achieve orgasm. My patients run the gamut of that particular dysfunction, too, from the woman who has never had an orgasm in her life to the woman who did have orgasms at one time, but doesn't anymore.

Seeing the flood of material that's being printed on the subject—both in the professional and in the popular press—it's obvious that my situation as a doctor is by no means unique. The problem is a common one, and it can be serious.

However, if there's one thing I've discovered in my years as a doctor, it's that things are not always what they seem to be. Sometimes people don't understand what's going on as well as they think they do, and the problem they believe they have turns out to be completely different from the problem they really have. So when a woman comes to my office and says, "Doctor, I've never had an orgasm," that's when I start asking questions.

The first thing I ask her is usually something like, "What is your idea of an orgasm? What do you think an orgasm should be?" You'd be astonished at the answers I get! Sometimes they even astonish *me*. The plain fact is, many women who claim they don't have orgasms don't really know what an orgasm is. To rephrase an old saying, they don't know what they *think* they're missing! It's something they have to be taught. They actually have to learn to recognize an orgasm when they have one.

One patient told me she thought an orgasm should be the way her friend, Betty, described it. "When Betty has an orgasm, she wants to scream and she wants to scratch—she goes wild!"

Another patient told me that when her friend, Jane, has an orgasm, "She ejaculates just like a man." That's not actually true, of course. Women don't ejaculate. It sounds to me as though Jane is probably a woman of high sexual intensity and she lubricates profusely. When she has the vaginal contractions that are natural with orgasm, she may force the lubricant out of her vagina. The combination of the lubricant flow and the contractions could make it seem as if she's ejaculating.

Yet another patient told me that she had read somewhere that when a woman has an orgasm she sees rainbows and beautiful colors, she sees sparklers going and fireworks, and she hears bells ringing. That same woman also said, with a great deal of sadness, "I have never experienced any of that."

Well, she may never experience "any of that." She—and many other women—may never have any of the feelings or sensations that *supposedly* come with orgasm. Many women just never allow their emotions to get that wild. But those women may have been having their own kind of orgasms right along, without even knowing it.

A favorite question of mine to women who complain they don't have orgasm is, "How do you feel after you've made love, or a petting session, or whatever you're accustomed to having as a sexual contact with your partner? What do you feel like when you are all through? Are you content to curl up in his arms and relax, and maybe go to sleep?"

That last question is an important one, because if you feel content and you're happy and relaxed and you're ready to curl up and fall asleep after a sexual contact—you've had an orgasm. On the other hand, if a sexual encounter leaves you feeling restless and you are thinking, "I wish he wouldn't stop," then you have not had an orgasm.

If you're anything like most of my patients, you're probably saying, "That's all very good, but I'm talking about a *real* orgasm." Well, so am I. Does a woman who just feels kind of relaxed and not restless after intercourse have a real orgasm? Of course she does. Very much so, in fact. An orgasm doesn't have to be an all-out "bell-ringer" to be a real orgasm. Many women never have a bell-ringer in their lives. But they have plenty of highly satisfactory, "real" orgasms. Orgasms differ from person to person. That's a basic fact.

Unfortunately, there's an emotional trap with orgasms that is very easy to fall into—allowing yourself to believe that another kind of orgasm is "better" than the kind you have. Believing that is nonsense. The kind of orgasm you have is the right kind for you. Be happy with what you have. If you start searching for the perfect orgasm, you're going to be sadly disappointed. I've told you before that you can't will an orgasm. Not only that, you can't will the kind of orgasm you want to have, either. If you want to increase the excitement and pleasure of your orgasms, the best thing you can do is learn to let yourself go a little more, relax a little more, and be a little more open with your emotions. That may take some practice.

One of the goals of people who are looking for the so-called "perfect" orgasm is the one known as "simultaneous" orgasm. If you believe a lot of things you read in magazines and books today, there's something wrong with you if you don't have simultaneous orgasm. Let me tell you, the myth—and I mean myth—that everyone should strive for simultaneous orgasm has been one of the chief offenders in producing sexual dysfunction.

One thing that makes it such a dangerous goal is that simultaneous orgasm is the exception rather than the rule. If a man is well trained to control himself and knows how to hold back his ejaculation until the woman is ready to have orgasm, the couple can have simultaneous orgasm. Of course, the odds are considerably better if the woman is multi-orgasmic.

There are a lot of people who don't even think simultaneous orgasm is all that great. They say there is no real sharing of the partner's orgasm because you are too busy having your own. They have a point. There is a special kind of joy in being aware of your partner having an orgasm, and then knowing that your partner is also aware of yours when you have it.

People who are well-adjusted sexually tend to accept whatever is the norm for them. If your norm is simultaneous orgasm, that's wonderful. But if that isn't your norm, then get the most out of what you've got instead of trying to find what you think you are missing.

We've discovered the fact that many women who think they don't have orgasm actually do—but that's not the whole picture. A lot of women who think they don't have orgasms are absolutely right—they don't!

One of the simplest and most common reasons for a woman not having an orgasm is that she just can't relax. Tension— even slight tension—is a great killer of sensation. Sometimes having a drink or two can be exactly the right thing to bring on relaxation. Another way to achieve relaxation is to use the massaging techniques I talked about in the chapter on specific male problems. In that chapter, the massage was used to help awaken sexual feelings—but it is always a very effective way to bring on relaxation.

The techniques of massage are the same for you as they are for the man. The difference is that this time the emphasis is on awakening your eroticism, on getting you aroused. So the first consideration has to be your feelings and your excitement. No matter how excited your partner gets and how much he wants to complete the act, everything must wait until *you* are ready. And even if you should want to, don't do it until you get to the same stage in the massage that it was allowed for the man.

That means you are going to have to be a little selfish, concentrate only on *your* feelings and disregard your partner's needs for the time being. You see, we're trying to do the same thing for you that we did for the man in the last chapter—take away the need to perform. The way a woman "performs" is by telling herself she must have an orgasm. At this point I want you to forget all about having an orgasm. Just concentrate on feeling good. The important thing is to relax enough to let yourself get past whatever barrier it is that keeps you from letting go completely enough to have an orgasm.

A lot of times, people will say, "I need a change of scene," almost as if it were a joke. The concept may be an old one by now, and even something of a cliché—but it really does work. A vacation or a weekend out of town can do wonders for you by removing you physically from the sources of your tensions.

Even having sex at a different time of day from your usual can have a relaxing effect.

Ordinary tension is the most common reason for a woman not having an orgasm, but it's by no means the only one. A primary cause of a woman's failure to have orgasm is marital discord. It's easy to see why. You can't relax and go all out with a man you are unhappy with. When you are having problems with one another, you don't feel like making love to one another. You don't feel like letting go of your emotions.

And another thing—if you squabble with him all the time, you're sure not going to want to give him the satisfaction of showing him you can still be excited by him.

Sexuality may be the original double-edged sword. If you are having marital troubles, those troubles are going to cause you problems in your sex life. But it works both ways. Problems you have with sex can be all it takes to get your marriage (or your relationship) in trouble.

All too often when that kind of trouble starts, many women use sex as a weapon. Let's be fair about it—men do that too. I can't tell you how dangerous that is. There just aren't too many things I can think of that are more certain to ruin a relationship than using sex as a weapon.

You never really get away with anything when you do that, you know. Very soon, it's going to be perfectly obvious to your partner exactly what you are doing. That's true whether you do it consciously or not. Whatever you do to use sex as a weapon, your partner is going to know it is because of the discord between you. And your partner is going to resent it. Getting over anger is one thing, but getting over resentment is many, many times harder!

As I've said, whenever I see a couple whose sexual problems are complicated by marital discord, I insist they go to a marriage counselor and get those problems ironed out first. There is no way I can treat a sexual disorder successfully if the marriage itself is in bad shape.

I never like to see a couple go to bed angry with each other. If you've had a spat sometime during the day or just before you go to bed and that makes you move apart from each other instead of kissing each other good night, that only adds to whatever other problems you might be having. My suggestion is that one of you do a little cuddling to show the other, "Look, we've had a little argument, but I still love you and I want to be close to you." Believe me, that can go a long way toward diminishing or wiping out the anger completely.

What about women who have had orgasms in the past, but no longer do? It's been my experience that most of those women will say it is the fault of the husband. And the husband will generally agree he is to blame, and perhaps it happened because *he* was having sexual problems. He tried less often, and she gradually got used to it. He became afraid to try, and those fears had an emotional effect on her.

When they did have sex, he took her to the plateau stage, but couldn't get her past that. Maybe she got tired of being taken to the brink so often and reacted by consciously or unconsciously withholding her feelings to the point where she became non-orgasmic.

Here's a problem—and it's a fairly typical one. You have a man who has slowed down his sexual activity because he has become afraid of failure. Now his wife is still very much in love with him. She knows about his fears, and she doesn't encourage him to try anything because she doesn't want to see him shamed or embarrassed.

So the whole thing becomes a behavior pattern. The less they do anything, the less they want to do anything. They have sex less and less often, until finally they stop altogether.

In cases like that, the woman's problem is perhaps best dealt with by curing the man!

I'd like to tell you briefly about some other causes of sexual dysfunction in women. They are not as common, but they are generally more serious. One of those problems is vaginismus. I gave you an example in Chapter 5 of a patient of mine with a serious case of vaginismus, but I think it might be a good idea to discuss the condition a little more here.

Vaginismus is really a problem younger women have. In fact, when an older woman has it, chances are it's a problem she's had for a very long time. That's by no means a hard and fast rule, though. An older woman who has vaginismus might have gotten it because of a recent emotional trauma or physical injury.

The treatment is simple and consists of gradually dilating the opening of the vagina, either with special instruments or with your fingers. The dilators are similar to dildos, and each one in the set is slightly larger than the previous one. You start with the smallest, and you slowly build up to the point where you can insert the largest one without discomfort. If the doctor prefers, he will teach you how to get the same results using your fingers. Very often, the cure is a quick one. I've seen patients cured of the condition in four or five treatments. That's about all I want to say about the treatment. If you have more questions, don't be afraid to ask your doctor.

Learning to relax should take care of the problem. If a woman has vaginismus, that's usually the extent of the problem. She can respond in every other way. In other words, she can go through all four stages of sexual excitement and might even have earth-shaking orgasms. The only thing she can't stand is to have her vagina entered.

You might think that if a woman can get excited during foreplay to the point of lubricating, an orgasm is inevitable. Sorry, but that's not always true. Some women get excited enough for lubrication to take place, but they have no feeling or sensation at all during intercourse.

How can a woman get excited if she doesn't have any sensation? I didn't say she didn't have *any* sensation. I just said she didn't feel anything *during intercourse*. Most likely she has plenty of sensation in her clitoris. What has probably happened is she has developed a behavior pattern of not responding. She doesn't know that the inner walls of the vagina have no sensation, and because she expects to have sensation in this area, she feels deprived when she doesn't. Actually, the only two areas that are highly sensitive are the clitoral area and perhaps the first half-inch or so of the vaginal entrance—with most of the sensation in the external genitalia and the inner lips of the vagina.

How can such a woman be helped? For one thing, she should know that it is not necessary to have orgasm by what people consider the "usual" way—penis-in-vagina intercourse. Nothing says intercourse must be the only way you have orgasm. What you need to do is reeducate yourself—teach your body that it has plenty of other areas that will respond with pleasure to stimulation. The best way I can think of to do this is to follow the techniques for massage given earlier in this chapter and in the previous one.

Here's a kind of variation of that problem. One of my female patients was able to get excited to the point of lubrication, take that excitement right up to the plateau stage, and then—nothing. Every time she had intercourse she would get right up to the final step, but she would not take that last step to orgasm.

What made her unable to do that? Finding the answer wasn't easy. It took some fairly close questioning to get to the cause of the problem. She held back her orgasms because she didn't want to give in to her husband. She didn't want her husband to think he had enough power over her to make her lose control of herself the way she would if she had an orgasm. Another—and more obvious—reason might have been that she was taught all her life that she was not supposed to enjoy intercourse. She may have been taught that intercourse is strictly for procreation, never for recreation. Or just for men's pleasure, never women's. She may have been taught to be a tool of her husband and just to do her duty.

It's really sad to see women denying themselves healthy, normal pleasures they are entitled to have because they've had those ideas from the Dark Ages drummed into them.

The most serious kind of sexual disorder is what we call "primary sexual dysfunction." That, as I have mentioned before, means the woman has never been excited to the point where she has lubricated. It's on the same level of seriousness as the problem of a man who has never had an erection firm enough to penetrate the vagina.

Frankly, that particular problem is too serious for me to even attempt to deal with in a book of this kind. A woman who has never been excited at all must be helped psychologically. The problem is usually one that goes way back to childhood—with complex causes, and her inhibitions and blocks will most likely require a long period of psychotherapy.

Now you know something about the usual reasons you might not be having orgasms. This may, therefore, be a good time for me to throw in one of my little warnings. Because of recent public attention through books, and magazines, orgasm has become so important that all too often a woman will fake it so her partner will think he has satisfied her. Men do that, too, by the way. Very often an older man won't realize that he doesn't need to ejaculate, or he fears he won't be able to keep his erection long enough to do it, so he hurries the process along and pretends he has ejaculated.

If you or your partner are ever tempted to fake orgasm—don't do it! For a woman to fake an orgasm or for a man to pretend he has ejaculated is a bad idea. In most cases, neither partner is fooled for any length of time. That kind of deception—let's not sugar-coat it; it *is* deception—only makes it harder to achieve the kind of trust you need for a good sexual relationship. Besides, many women get a great deal of pleasure from the act itself, and it may not matter to them if they have an orgasm. The goal of sex is pleasure—and that's to be had with or without orgasm.

So if your partner asks you, be honest about it. If you haven't had an orgasm, don't be afraid to tell him so. A considerate lover will continue to manipulate you until he does get you to orgasm. However, your responses are slowed as you get older, so you are going to take longer to reach your orgasm. If your partner ejaculates before you do have your orgasm, that could be a problem. Once an older man ejaculates, he becomes flaccid very quickly and he'll slip right out.

Remember one thing, though—his fingers don't get flaccid. There's no reason he can't continue by manipulating you to orgasm.

Bear in mind that there's an ego problem involved, so if you tell your partner you haven't had an orgasm, be a little careful about how you phrase it. The wrong tone of voice could make your answer sound like you're blaming him for it. You could say something like, "Not yet, but keep it up and I'll probably get there."

Here are some final thoughts on orgasm. Nobody is responsible for your sexual satisfaction. You are responsible for your own feelings, and you are the master of your own feelings. It's not your partner's responsibility to make you orgasmic, nor is it your responsibility to make him orgasmic. In the process of relaxation and enjoying each other, you reach the pinnacle of satisfaction on your own. You are responsible for your own reactions.

Chapter 14:
SEXUALLY TRANSMITTED DISEASES

Whenever I give a talk anywhere, I always try to take time to answer questions from the audience. Without fail, there will be questions about venereal disease. That's what I'd like to talk to you about now. It's not a pleasant subject, I know, and it might be something that causes you a lot of anxiety—but it's something that has to be talked about because it's something that could happen to you.

By the way, you'll notice the title of this chapter refers to "Sexually Transmitted Disease," STD, which is what the medical profession is calling venereal disease now. It's a much more accurate title than the old one. Personally, I think it sounds less threatening, too.

The first thing you want to know about STD is, "Can I catch one at my age?" I'm sorry to have to tell you, yes, you can. STD is no respecter of age or social status.

Even in this liberated day and age, the idea of acquiring a sexually transmitted disease has an impact that shocks the emotions. It affects your feeling of security, it affects your feeling of trust for your partner. A not unusual reaction is, "How could it happen to me? I'm so ashamed I don't know how I can face even my doctor." That sense of shame, unfortunately, does keep a lot of people from seeking treatment until the disease has taken firm hold, and in some cases until it's too late to be treated at all.

Take something as simple as a yeast infection. Women get yeast infections all the time, and they treat it as something to be gotten rid of and then forgotten. They don't anguish over it, but treat it just like any other malady. Many of you women reading this now have had that experience, I'm sure. But let it be known that one of the ways yeast infections can be transmitted is by sexual intercourse, and you have a whole new situation. What was ordinary before is now a matter of shame and embarrassment, and it somehow turns into a subject that can't be talked about. Why? Because people still have too many funny ideas about sex, that's why.

A prominent public health official once said, "If we could convince people that venereal disease was caught from toilet seats, or from any other way but sexual contact, we could wipe it out almost literally overnight." He's not exaggerating too much, you know. If we could learn to regard an STD as no worse than a bad head cold, we could finally get rid of it once and for all.

Why don't we backtrack now, and talk about some of the different forms of STD. When I was in medical school back in the thirties, we only knew of five venereal diseases—gonorrhea, syphilis, chancroid and a couple of others that were fairly rare. Now we know there are closer to twenty. You might wonder how it is that now we have about twenty, but in the old days we managed to get along with only five! In the old days, we didn't know that the rest of those now on the list could be transmitted sexually. We knew about the diseases, for the most part, but not enough about how people got them.

The yeast infection I just mentioned is a good example. We've known for a long time that a woman could get it as an indirect result of taking antibiotics. That's because the antibiotics kill the organisms which inhibit the growth of the yeast. With nothing to stop it, the yeast can flourish. Now we know she can pick it up from sexual contact as well.

Even though there have been many changes in the listing and classification of those diseases, the two big ones are still with us and going stronger than ever. I refer, of course, to gonorrhea and syphilis.

The first symptom of gonorrhea in a man is a discharge or drip of pus from the urethra. That's easy enough to spot, because men don't usually have that kind of discharge, so they'll notice the change immediately. A woman with gonorrhea may have a day or two of burning or itching around her vagina, and she may have some discharge. However, there are a couple of kickers. First of all, a woman's symptoms might pass completely unnoticed—a discharge is not that unusual a thing for a woman. Which means she could have the disease and be completely unaware of it until she is told by someone she has had sex with who contracted it from her.

The second thing is, about 15 percent of all the men who contract gonorrhea don't show any symptoms. But they are still carriers and can pass it on to others.

The second of the two best-known STD's, syphilis, has also been around awhile. It has been referred to as the greatest mimic of all diseases. It can attack anywhere, and it can produce symptoms of any kind of disease. What makes it so treacherous is the first symptoms can occur anywhere from ten to ninety days after contact.

The first sign of syphilis is a sore called a chancre. A chancre can range in size from a tiny pimple to an ulcer the size of a quarter. It's painless, and it disappears in two or three weeks whether you treat it or not. The chancre appears at whatever point the syphilis organism enters the body. That won't necessarily be on the genitals or anywhere near them. The chancre could turn up on the mouth or on an open sore—both common sites of infection.

The second stage of syphilis consists of a rash, which is hard to identify for what it is because it looks like any other rash. Again, even if you don't treat it, this symptom will go away with time. After that, many years could go by before the final effects of the third and final stages are felt. The final stage attacks the central nervous system.

Treatments for syphilis and gonorrhea were pretty horrible in the old days, but that's no longer the case. Cures that used to take weeks or even years are now handled in one or two visits to the doctor for gonorrhea, and seven to twelve daily visits for syphilis. Most of the time now, it's as easy to knock out those diseases as it is to contract them.

All right, it's easy for you to contract those diseases. How likely is it that you will? I'd have to say the chances are much higher than they used to be. No matter how careful you are, you can't be sure that everyone else is as careful. In this day of more liberal morality and more open views on sex, it is more than ever possible that young and sexually active women will be attracted to older men. The reverse is also true, by the way. Of course, that can increase the chances of getting a disease. So you might be thinking, "I'll stay away from young people, and I'll be okay. I'll just do it with people my own age."

I wish I could tell you, "Do that, and all your worries are over," but I can't. There is always the chance that your partner has had contact with somebody with the disease, which that person caught from a contact who caught it from another contact who . . . well, I think you get the idea. It's kind of like the story of the old-timer who liked to brag, "I shook the hand of a man who shook the hand of a man who shook the hand of a man who shook the hand of a man who shook the hand of a man who shook the hand of Abraham Lincoln!"

I don't want to give you the complete medical school course in gonorrhea and syphilis. I do, however, want you to be aware of them, and be aware that they can take you by surprise. The symptoms are often so subtle you can easily miss them completely. If you have been following my advice about becoming more and more aware of your body, you are going to be in a good position to spot anything that might be irregular and go to a doctor with the problem. It's also essential for you to see a doctor if you have had a sexual contact with someone you aren't sure about. Please don't neglect any of those signs of irregularity or any misgivings you might have about a sexual partner. The consequences can be too serious.

For example, an untreated case of gonorrhea in either a man or a woman can produce very serious complications by extending backward into the vital organs. It can destroy normal, necessary body functions, and cause a lot of pain and physical hardship.

What I'm asking you to do is *please* not rule out the possibility that something wrong with you might be an STD. Go to a doctor. Let the doctor rule out the possibility.

The important thing to remember is that it is not a shameful or embarrassing thing for a doctor or social worker to hear you have contracted an STD. We know there is a lot of it around, and we know it is common to all kinds of people and all social classes. Believe me, if you come in with one, your doctor is not going to treat you like a tramp or a bum for catching such a nasty thing. Be assured that most of us have seen those conditions many, many times, and we know they are innocently acquired in most instances. No embarrassing questions will be asked of you. If you come in with a disease in the early stages, you'll probably find your doctor is happy about your showing so much common sense. And let me tell you from my own experience as a doctor, you make your doctor's job easier—and you make the cure a lot easier on yourself.

So don't let the fear of contracting a disease keep you from enjoying your sexuality to the fullest. The best precautions you can take involve nothing more than common sense. The most important part of that is good hygiene. Wash yourself carefully, keep your body, your clothing and your bed linens clean. Try to be selective in your choice of sexual partners. You shouldn't have too much to worry about.

There are still some things I want to say about STD's in general, but it might be a good idea to give you a little reassurance. Syphilis and gonorrhea are dangerous and scary, and it's important for you to know about them so you can protect yourself. I just don't want to leave you thinking you are a sure bet to get one of them. That's simply not the case. If I were to give you tips on safe driving, would that mean I thought you were likely to have an accident? Of course not! The same applies to those STD's. Chances are you'll never get one—especially if you use common sense and follow the guide lines I've given you.

Now, what about the other kinds of STD? They are

relatively innocuous, and hardly any of them have the potential for the kind of serious complications that can develop with syphilis and gonorrhea. As I mentioned earlier, many of them can be picked up by non-sexual contact.

Three kinds of STD I'd like to mention specifically involve women. They are trichomonas vaginalis, yeast infections, and hemophilus vaginalis. Until fairly recently, they were not thought to be sexually transmitted, though they are as old as the history of medicine. All three of them produce vaginal discharges.

Trichomonas is caused by a parasite. There are millions of them swarming around in the discharge, which produces an intense itching. The discharge itself is yellow, frothy, and very foul-smelling. In the old days, we didn't have too much trouble curing it, though the methods we used were rather cruel. We scrubbed the women with harsh soaps, prescribed harsh and irritating douches and ointments. I remember sometimes we'd scrub a woman with tinctured green soap, and she'd hardly be able to walk out of the office, she was so sore. The difficulty was keeping them cured, because we didn't know it was a sexually transmittable disease. Men can pass it on and never know they have it.

Once we discovered that men could carry it, we began to make some headway against it. The cure turned out to be simple—all we had to do was keep the man from having direct contact with the woman. He could have intercourse, but he had to use a condom. The organism then died a natural death in the man, because it couldn't survive in the acid environment of the urine. That part was easy, but the treatment for the woman was as rough as ever, until a drug was developed that knocked the organism right out. The drug is Flagyl, and is available with a doctor's prescription. It is taken by both partners orally for seven to ten days.

The yeast infection is another very common condition. The discharge is heavier and white, with a paste-like consistency. There is considerable itching, but no odor. One of the reasons yeast infections are so common these days is the increased use of antibiotics. Antibiotics destroy the organisms that keep the yeast organisms in check, and so they can flourish. Yeast infection is not as easily transmitted by sexual contact as some other conditions, but it frequently does occur that way. It's a relatively difficult condition to treat because it recurs so frequently. There are many treatments for it, and hardly a year can go by without a new cure coming on the market.

The best precaution I can suggest is for both you and your partner to wash carefully both before and after intercourse.

Hemophyllis vaginalis has a thin, watery discharge, with an odor. It's a fairly common condition, and it's easy to cure. Like the others, it does come back, and also like the other two, there are no serious complications. Very few women avoid having one or more of these infections during their lifetimes.

Now let's talk about something that attacks—and I mean that literally—both men and women. I mean head lice, body lice, and the infamous pubic lice, or crabs. They can be picked up in many ways. You can get them from body contact, from wearing the clothing of someone who has them, from contact with the bedclothes of a victim. If you should be unlucky enough to catch any of these or other mite diseases, let your doctor direct the treatment. Although mite diseases are easy to cure, you could overtreat it and make it worse.

You know, I could go on for a long time about this, but I don't think you need to know everything about the different types of STD. I'd like to reassure you, however, that they generally will not hit you any harder or be any more difficult to cure just because you are older. And remember, while many of those diseases and infections can be transmitted sexually, they don't necessarily start that way. What happens is they often start out some other way and then continue back and forth through sexual contact.

I've had many an irate husband come into my office and say something like, "Hey, what the hell is going on here? My wife catches something, and now I have to be careful. What is it she's got that I have to be careful about? What did she pick up?" And very often he wonders, "Am I being indirectly accused of bringing something home? I've been a faithful husband, and we've had a fine relationship."

So I have to explain to him how the antibiotic she was taking a few weeks before caused a yeast infection, and we are trying to make the cure take by keeping them from passing the organism back and forth like a tennis ball.

There's no reason a couple should have any problems over most of the STD's they are likely to encounter. But what if you should pick up one of the biggies? What if you get syphilis or gonorrhea and expose your partner? That's a problem, and not a very pleasant one, I'm afraid. Sometimes if you know you've caught a dose and you avoid contact with your partner, you can be cured and he or she could never know the difference. If you've had contact, that's another story. Your partner is going to have to know. It's a nice fantasy to think your doctor can get your partner into the office with some excuse that will hide the real reason, but things don't usually work out that smoothly. Fooling people who know you well is never easy.

Really, the best thing you can do is be honest about it. Tell your partner what you have picked up and get him or her in for treatment as fast as possible. Yes, you are likely to have a hell of a rough time over it. Your partner may be understanding, but you can hardly expect to be congratulated. Go to a counselor or therapist, if necessary; just don't let a serious disease fester undetected until your partner becomes seriously ill and never knows why. No matter how hard it is, be honest.

Chapter 15:
GETTING BACK INTO THE SWING OF THINGS

I know there are many of you reading this book who are widows and widowers. And I also know many of you are in good health and yet you feel totally indifferent to anything around you—especially sex. Your problem is not an uncommon one. What has happened to you is that you have simply lost touch with your own sexuality.

That kind of thing happens for a lot of reasons. You may never have gotten over the loss of your spouse, for example. Or there may have been other things that have depressed you, and the depression deepened to the point where you couldn't shake it. Depression is a powerful thing. Once you get into a depression, you tend to withdraw into a shell and stay away from your old friends—particularly your old friends who are married.

Depression is something you've got to get yourself out of, or it can wreck you. So if you are depressed, don't stay in your shell—get out of it. If you can't do it by yourself, don't wait until it gets bad enough to make you helpless—get to your family doctor, who will sit and talk to you and try to find out what made you so depressed and how long the condition has lasted. If he can't help you, he will refer you to someone who can.

Depression, of course, is a disease—a serious disease. It's an illness, and in most cases it is a cause of sexual dysfunction. It can take months and months of good psychotherapy to break through. The treatment will vary with the individual, of course, and it will depend on how long the person has been depressed and how much the person has been removed from social contact. That's as true for the young as it is for the old—especially for the older people who think they have outlived their usefulness.

The problem of people who think they have outlived their usefulness is a heartbreaking one. I have seen the results of that attitude too many times in my life. I have seen many elderly men and women who have been deserted by their children or other family members because they could no longer take care of themselves. Those older people became slovenly in appearance and didn't keep themselves clean enough; they didn't eat the proper foods or get enough exercise to keep themselves healthy. When their condition got bad enough, their children put them in a nursing home and gave up on them. Here many of them may become almost complete vegetables.

Anxiety, fear, and depression are probably the greatest factors in producing senility and certainly affect sexual vigor, libido, and activity. That's why the earlier you try to do something about that depression, the easier it is going to be to cure.

Let's talk about senility for a moment. Most of the people who are supposedly senile are not that way because their brains have degenerated for lack of blood supply—caused by diseased arteries not providing enough blood to the brain. No, most of those people are called senile because they just went into a state of depression and they were never brought out of it. That happened either because they didn't want to be brought out of it or because other people gave up on them too easily and they took the easy way out and gave up on themselves.

There have been some recent experiments dealing with senility. The researchers have taken people in nursing homes who were regarded as being hopelessly senile—at what is called the "vegetable" stage—and forced them little by little to come out of their shells.

The idea was to make the old people feel wanted. Most of them had been treated like little children and pampered like little children. The object of the project was to make them interested in life and in things around them, and make them feel important and needed again. One of the ways that was accomplished was to teach the older people to read and write again, show them pictures, and generally retrain and re-educate them. The researchers did everything they could think of to awaken those brains that had been put to sleep by inactivity, not by disease. Has the program been successful? You bet it has. Once you get the brain to start working, it tends to continue, and not only that—it tends to want more.

Retirement can be a tricky thing for an older person. Some people look forward to it, and they thrive on it when it comes. But all too often, retirement means compulsory retirement—and that usually means retirement before you are ready for it. The idea of retirement at a specific age is, I think, one of the worst things in the world that can happen to people. Our senior population is growing every year, and our society contains a higher and higher percentage of older individuals. I'm sure many of you have seen your friends slowly deteriorate and even die after being forced to retire.

I know many teaching doctors who were forced to retire because they had reached the age limit for their universities—even though they were bright and alert and contributing great things to the literature of medicine. Most die within two years of the forced retirement age.

Sure, the retirement laws exist for many reasons, some beneficial. We retire the person who has lost his interest and his enthusiasm, who has lost his memory, and who isn't aware he's been failing. But it is cruel to the others—people who are still active and who are still able to perform. And I think that's the greatest single cause of depression in our older folks today.

I have a patient who was a brilliant man, fluent in eight languages. He worked for a large bank that handled a good deal of foreign business, so he was very valuable to them. Well, because he was so good at his job and so valuable, they let him work long past the compulsory retirement age of sixty-five. Then, unfortunately, others in the bank made an issue of his age—he was seventy-one at that time—and the bank had to let him go. That was a real blow to him. One day he was important and useful, the next day he was an unemployed old man of seventy-one who happened to speak a lot of languages.

He was so shocked emotionally that he pulled a mental shell around himself and started to go downhill in a hell of a hurry. No amount of encouragement did anything for him. There were so many things I tried to get him involved in, but nothing worked. I put him in touch with a couple of community organizations. One of them asked him to use his language ability to read and write letters for people whose English was poor; the other asked him to help with their office work. He turned them both down because he considered the tasks unimportant and menial.

The sad thing is that what *he* considered unimportant was very important to the people he would have been helping. Nobody could get him interested in anything, and now he's slowly but surely becoming a helpless cripple. He barely walks; he won't look at TV, isn't interested in a newspaper—and this is a man who had been an avid reader.

But in spite of all the reasons forced retirement is a bad idea, society still compels people to retire at a certain age, no matter what they are capable of doing. However, recent legislation has already begun to strike down that kind of outmoded practice. It's criminal how often someone is shoved aside who still has plenty on the ball, who still has a lot to offer society. These people are useful, and it's a real boost to society when older people continue to maintain an interest in their fields, or in other fields, and continue to produce useful, valuable information for society in general, and produce to their fullest capacities.

I've gotten a lot of pleasure out of the fact that a well-known medical school raised itself to the front ranks by simply hiring the excellent—and often famous—teachers who had been forced into retirement by less enlightened schools.

Now with all this, don't get the idea that I'm telling you a retired person has to make significant contributions to the world to keep from getting depressed. As long as you feel *useful* in some way, no matter how small, that's all you need.

Not very long ago, I was on the panel of a seminar on the problems of aging. Among the things we discussed were how to prevent aging and what could be done to prevent senility. The consensus of opinion was that the cure was not going to be found in any drug or medicine. The way to combat problems of senility was to keep the mind active, read, join in group discussions, attend lectures and concerts and the theatre. In short, do everything you can to keep yourself from becoming mentally dull.

That all comes down to one thing, doesn't it? It means getting back into the swing of things. How do you get back into the swing of things? Well, as I said in the beginning of this chapter, you have to get out and start meeting people.

Meeting people is a lot easier these days than it used to be. Organizations of every kind are falling all over themselves to keep the "senior citizens" happy. There are hundreds of Golden Age groups available today, in churches, synagogues, in clubs, in social welfare agencies, and most of those groups are literally humming with activities. That, of course, is where you are going to learn to go out in society again, to talk to people and to meet people.

One of my patients is a seventy-eight-year-old widow who developed Parkinson's disease. Well, with the new medicines we now have we were able to help her. She has started going to church groups, and she talks now about the dances she goes to and how well she enjoys dancing and how many boyfriends she has. She told me, "Not that I bring them home with me or that I go to their homes, but we have a lot of fun when we go to those parties that are given in the churches."

Let me tell you about a man from my old neighborhood in Chicago who I think really understands the idea of keeping young. I'll call him Max. One day I ran into him when I was out mailing a letter, and we stopped by the mailbox to chat. We got to talking about keeping young, and Max (who was seventy-nine at the time) said to me, "I'm young. If you want to see old, I'll show you old," and he pointed down the street to a man shuffling slowly toward us. "He's six years younger than me, would you believe it? Every day he takes the same walk. From his apartment building to this corner. And from that block and a half, he has to lean for two minutes on the mailbox here so he can get his wind back for the return trip." As the man came up to the mailbox, Max asked him, "Why do you take the same walk every day? Why not go down the street to the library someday, look up the town where you were born and find out as much as you can about it?" The man looked at Max in disgust and said, "Ah, I know all that stuff already."

After he was gone, Max said to me, "You see, he's old. He let himself get old."

Another thing about Max. He had just started out in a new career as an actor. He had done *The Sunshine Boys* in summer stock, and he was complaining because he had to join Actors Equity (the professional actors' union). Well, of course, it was really obvious how proud he was of himself. He said he was talking to a friend about his acting, and his friend said, "Max, you're crazy in the head, starting something like this at your age. What do you think you can do?" So Max told him, "I don't know, but I'm sure as hell going to try to find out. I'm giving myself five years to make it." At seventy-nine, mind you.

Naturally, I asked him what he would consider "making it." You know what he said? His goal—by age eighty-four—is a TV series of his own!

A good way to keep yourself mentally active is to associate with younger people. I feel that mixing with younger people is a very important thing. My own mother was lucky that way. She didn't consider herself old, and she was very mentally alert. She was still able to live with her children, and we brought our young friends around. She tried to stay up on the events of the day so she could join in the conversations of the younger crowd.

The problem of getting back into the swing of things is more difficult for a woman than it is for a man. Most men, except those who are very depressed or very introverted, find it fairly easy to get back into the world, to rediscover people, places, and pace. One reason men can get back into circulation somewhat more easily than most women is that they are usually more accustomed to being out in the world to begin with. They're used to meeting people. Another reason is that the older women so far outnumber them that even a man who is not particularly attractive is likely to find himself being approached by women.

But once you meet a few people, I'm sure you can always find somebody you can ask to go places with you. And that goes for both sexes. A man should have no problem at all asking a woman to go to the theatre with him. And women, too, who have theatre tickets will find there is no real problem at all about calling a gentleman friend to say, "Look, I have two tickets to such-and-such a show. Would you like to go with me?" Most men will jump at the opportunity. And who knows what might come from that first encounter.

In our culture, older women seem to socialize more often with other women. They play cards and go to the theatre together. Part of the reason for that is the dearth of men. Women in the age group we're talking about outnumber men by about five to one, so it's often a necessity for women to find companionship among themselves. They take care of themselves pretty well, too, because people who are out with other people don't want to look sloppy. Women are generally brought up to be a little more self-reliant than men are, so they can often take care of themselves better when they are alone.

Women can be perfectly happy with female companionship. You very often will see groups of women at theatres, groups of women going to picnics, groups of women joining clubs. In fact, the audiences at my lectures are predominantly women.

Men, of course, can join clubs, and some of the best are in gyms. They join the calisthenics classes. There are Golden Age groups which include both men and women, but I've found that men don't go for them quite as much as women do. You won't find groups of men going to the theatre, but groups of women sitting in a whole row of a theatre together is a common sight.

If you women are so outnumbered and it's so much harder for you to get back into things socially, what can you do? You can take the lead, that's what you can do. Women today—even older women—are breaking down that old taboo against women being the aggressor in a relationship. Nowadays it's likely to be the woman who says hello first, and it's likely to be the woman who asks the man to dance. While you're dancing with him, what's wrong with starting a conversation? You might even ask him, "How long has it been since you've had a good home-cooked meal?"

Personally, I think it's delightful for a woman to be a little aggressive with a man. Now, by aggressive, I don't mean you should pounce on a man and say, "I need you, I want you, let's go to my room!" But do at least be aggressive to the point of starting a conversation with a man. Many a shy man will really welcome a woman making the first move. You'll be amazed at how quickly you carry on from there.

We're starting to get into an area that is a little bit tricky for some people, so maybe it would be a good idea for me to lay it all out now and get it over with. One of the things you're probably going to end up doing is dating. Did your stomach just do a little flip? I know the feeling. It's funny, but when I talked about the subject with some friends of mine, I got that reaction, too. In fact, one of them told me, "Joe, when you tell me I should start having sex again at my age (he's sixty-eight), I think that's fine and I want to hear more about it. But when you tell me I should start dating again at my age—frankly, it scares hell out of me!"

I don't know what it is, but I went through the same thing when I started dating after my first wife died. Maybe the fact that it's so public has something to do with it. You go on a date, and you're out where other people can see you. You start to think, "They know I'm not married to this woman. They know I'm out on a date with her, just like a kid. I feel like a total jackass."

Dating is a skill, and it's a skill you can easily lose. A young patient of mine had an experience which points that up: "I went out with a married man once," she said. "He'd only been married for about two years, but when he drove me home, he said, 'I'm supposed to walk you to the door now, aren't I?' This was a young guy, and he had already lost the basic skills of dating."

I would assume that many of you reading this have not

dated since you were very young. If you are a widow or a widower, you have spent years with someone and gotten used to that, and now you have to try to establish a new relationship from scratch. Older people know how to act with each other in a social situation, and a sexual situation, but not in a dating situation.

Suppose a man and a woman run into each other at a meeting of some kind, and afterward the man says, "Why don't we stop for a cup of coffee?" There will be no pressure, and they will probably both stay relaxed and have a good time. But take the same two people, the same meeting, and the man says, "Would you go to a movie with me Friday night?" . . . you've got a completely different situation. Now you've got social pressure. Each of them is going to start worrying about making an impression on the other. There will be anxieties about what to wear, what to say, will he or she like me? By the time Friday rolls around, both of them will be basket cases.

The friend I mentioned earlier who was so scared of the idea of dating finally calmed down enough to ask me, "All right, suppose I did ask somebody out on a date. What can we do? I mean you don't just ask a woman to have a date with you—you ask her if she would like to do thus and so. What's a good thus and so for a first date?"

A good question, and one that I'm asked often by my patients. I think a nice way to start off is to go out to dinner. Movies are great for young kids, because they eliminate the need for a lot of talking. I think older people like to talk, though, and a nice dinner is a good time to do that. You'll have a better chance to get acquainted, to find out about each other. In fact, any activity that allows you to relax and talk is a good one for the first date. You could go to a zoo, a flower show, an art exhibit, a museum—or just a walk in the park. Sit on a bench and watch the other people and talk; that's a fine first date. You might also consider how you met the person. You might want to do something related to an activity at which you met.

I'm sure you women are aware that your dates are likely to make passes at you. How do you handle them? First of all, don't be alarmed if it happens, because it probably will. A lot of men have been conditioned to believe that any woman, especially one who's been a widow for a long time, has to be a sure thing. He's likely to feel he's doing you a favor by offering to show you a good time in bed. Never feel you have to prove anything to anyone about your sexuality. You don't have to go to bed with anyone if you don't want to. If a man doesn't appeal to you, by all means turn him down. And if you're not sure how you feel, being turned down might make him more interested the next time.

It works both ways, you know. You men are quite likely to find a woman making pretty straightforward sexual approaches to you. If she invites you to come in and you aren't ready to get involved, all you have to do is make an excuse. For me it was easy. All I ever had to say was, "I'd love to, but I can't. I have early surgery tomorrow." If you're retired, tell her you have to get up early to take your grandchildren somewhere.

Now when you are a little bit more sure of yourself, a little bit more secure, you might want to give in a little bit. Start out, of course, with what you think is maybe gentle petting, and progress from there if you want to. But that's up to you. I'd like to continue with the problems a woman is likely to have for a while. If you have abstained from sex for a long time, whatever the reason, you may find it difficult to return to sexuality. I'd like to refer you back to the chapter on masturbation. Masturbation is a great way to reactivate and restimulate your sexual vigor. As I've said before, it's perfectly normal, perfectly legitimate. It's also a good way to relieve the tensions that go along with inhibitions, and reawaken the desire, perhaps, to actively look for another sexual partner.

You men, on the other hand, have to be reminded that if you have abstained for a long time, it isn't necessarily because of any loss of sexual power. If you wake up with an erection in the morning from time to time, as I've said, that's all the proof you need that everything is still working all right.

As I've said many times before, the fear of impotence is the greatest single cause of impotence. Just bear in mind that if you have abstained from sex for a long time, the first attempt is likely to be a failure. That's to be expected, even if the equipment is in basically good working order.

If you fail in your first encounter after a long period of

abstinence, you shouldn't feel embarrassed, because as a general rule your partner will have had that experience with her husband long before he died. She sort of expects it, and may be very happy to just accept the foreplay and the petting that goes with it, and be perfectly content with the excitement you've aroused in her, for the time being. That's even more likely if she hasn't had sexual contact with a male for a long time.

What about the tendency of older men to go after younger women when they get back into circulation? Yes, that does happen a lot, and it's hard on the older woman because she feels she can't be as attractive to an older man as a younger woman can. But many a romance has started in a Golden Age group. I have several friends who are in social work with Golden Age groups, and they have attended many a wedding of couples who are about the same age—in many cases the woman was even older than the man. And they have found a great deal of happiness together.

Chapter 16:
THE ATTITUDES OF OTHERS, AND SOME ODDS AND ENDS

One of the strongest influences on anyone, no matter what the age, social standing or education, is what other people think. Sometimes it goes even beyond that. Sometimes the deciding factor isn't what people do think, it's what they might be going to think. Maybe it ought not to matter, but of course, in honesty, it does. I'm sure you don't have to be told how the opinions of others can influence us on such a sensitive subject as sex. And if "public opinion" can influence us about sex generally, think how much effect its going to have on the idea of sex for older people.

Attitudes are changing, but most of the change seems to be on the part of the older people themselves. The new sexual freedom we have today has made a real impact on the sexuality of the aged. Anytime I need proof of that, all I have to do is look at the number of articles and pamphlets that have been written on the subject. Another good sign that it's true is the crowds I draw whenever I speak on the subject.

Yes, the older people seem to me to be eager to join in the sexual revolution, and another small sign of that is the fact that you are reading this book. But be that as it may, there are still far too many people running around with mid-Victorian ideas about sex—particularly sex for older people.

There was an article in *Psychology Today* magazine not long ago which gave the results of a poll of college students about their parents' sexual habits. I was stunned by what I read. If those young people were correct, their parents are living lives of sexual abstinence that would do a convent or a monastery proud. Oh, I think the youngsters realize their parents occasionally have intercourse. But I don't think they believe it happens very often, or that such dalliance is conducted with much imagination. For example, most of them seemed to discount entirely the possibility that their own parents might indulge in something like oral sex.

Children tend to have some strange ideas about their parents and sex. They simply cannot believe that their parents do "such things." "Not *my* parents," they say. "After all, they're grandparents now; they've got *grandchildren,* for Pete's sake, and I think they're much too old to think about such silly things as sex."

Children must be taught to understand that sexuality does exist in the elderly. They are fortunate, indeed, if they have parents who are sexually interested in each other, because it is an indication that the parents are very much in love with each other and don't take each other for granted. They are people who still have an intimate, affectionate, sympathetic, and understanding life together.

How can older people cope with the attitudes of their children? Well, it isn't easy. There isn't much the elderly couple themselves can do, but there sure is a lot that can be done by educators. There are articles on just about every aspect of sexuality you can imagine. The trouble is, more of them should be focused on changing the attitudes of younger people toward their elders.

For example, the article in *Psychology Today* that I mentioned indicated very strongly that awareness of the sexuality of older people has actually regressed since Kinsey's time.

I've had young people come to me and say, "My parents are acting like kids, and it's really embarrassing. You'd think they could get it on or something. They hold hands, they cuddle, they make jokes with each other about how sexy they are, things like that. Who do they think they're kidding?"

My response is, if they're not doing it to excess, if they're not making it very obvious in a tasteless way and all they're doing is what you would do in company—what's wrong with it? If you don't think your own behavior and the behavior of your peers is embarrassing, then you should be very proud of your parents. You should be very happy that your parents are still able to enjoy life and enjoy themselves. And, besides, what makes you so sure your parents don't still "get it on?"

One way you can handle the criticisms of your kids is with humor and with a sense of affection for each other. Here are some things you might say. Try one or two out, or maybe let them trigger some ideas of your own:

"The fact that your father and I have this kind of relationship is one of the big reasons we're able to take care of ourselves and leave you alone. But . . . if you don't want us to do this, we'll just stop and move in with you. Hey, that's not a bad deal. We can slop around all day and hang around, and you can take us places and entertain us."

"You mean *you* don't like doing it, and you're planning to give it up someday?"

"What year are *you* gonna stop?"

"Ahhh . . . you're worried about your inheritance! Okay, Sam, no more babies—for their sake."

"Don't you think you're going to be happier growing older if you know you don't have to give this up?"

A widow or a widower who decides to remarry has an entirely different problem. There the problem is not embarrassment, but jealousy and even fear. Jealousy over losing the affection and attention of a parent, and fear over the loss of inheritance. It's not uncommon for the children of a widower to worry if "that woman" is going to get all "their" money. They might fear that what their father doesn't spend foolishly in courtship he will leave to her when he dies, and they will be cut off. Or if it's a widow we're talking about, the kids might think, "What is she going to do with the money my father left her that we ought to be getting?"

In that kind of situation, any hostility by the children is usually more because of greed than because they really care if their parent has a sexual relationship or not. As soon as a widow or widower indicates an interest in marrying again, the children start in with the objections. From some of the things I've heard, they'll say almost anything, too.

In my opinion, who gets the inheritance is a practical problem, not an emotional one. Talk things over with a lawyer and get some ideas about the various ways it can be handled. The trick in a situation like that is to avoid letting the problem become an emotional one that comes between you and your children or between you and your partner. There's love and there's money; it's a pity to confuse them at this stage of your life.

Nursing homes have always made me very uncomfortable whenever I visited them as a doctor visiting a patient. I made a point of making as many visits as I could, because I know how my patients looked forward to them. Seeing me meant they hadn't been abandoned. They knew that at least I came regularly to see them and to talk to them, to cheer them up.

If I had my way about it, I'd set up nursing homes in an entirely different way from the way they are now. I'd make them more like retirement homes. For example, there's no need to have nurses and other employees running around in their uniforms in areas where the patients are ambulatory. Those people are there because there's no other place for them to be. They can take care of themselves, they feed themselves, they dress and undress themselves, and they can make their own beds, if necessary. The personnel in these areas should be dressed in regular clothes. There's no need to make the place look like a hospital.

One thing the nursing homes could do is provide more privacy for the individual, more freedom of action—and no dividing the men's section from the women's section. The homes should allow the intermingling of the sexes, but they should not allow the intermingling of relatively healthy people, independent and clear-minded, with people who are totally incapacitated and mentally deficient. There is nothing in the

The Attitudes of Others, and Some Odds and Ends 187

world that will make a well person deteriorate quicker than living with those who are totally deteriorated themselves.

Double beds should be provided for a husband and wife who are admitted together. I can see no reason in the world they should not be allowed to live in the same room.

The staffs of the nursing homes should be taught not to act so much as wardens who are constantly shaking their fingers and saying, "You shouldn't be doing that!" No, they should be taught to be considerate and smile at people.

A clergyman I know, a social worker who was in charge of a nursing home run by his church, was asked what he does when one of the staff reports seeing a resident entering the room of someone of the opposite sex. The director said, "I tell them to walk quietly, shut the door and say nothing, and if possible keep the biddies of the home from gossiping about the situation. Pretend you never saw it, and disregard the complaints that come in."

Those homes should provide areas that are pleasant where couples can sit quietly and hold hands without anybody pointing a finger at them. The homes don't have to be matchmakers, but they should make it easy for those people who can communicate with one another to do so. Many a love affair has started in a nursing home. I have seen them.

Fortunately, things are changing. Many institutions are being built which are like hotels. The people—male, female, singles, widows, widowers, and even married couples can live cheaply. They have their own apartments, and they share a common dining room where they can socialize and where activities are constantly going on for people who want them.

Most of all, these people should be surrounded by young people. Old people want to be near young people. They don't want to be with their peers only. No old person considers himself old if he's vigorous. The only way he will consider himself old is if he's relegated to a traditional old people's home. The staff and the people around them should be young. Not only young, though. They should have a particular interest in old people.

I think these institutions should make a habit of allowing children to visit—even if they are not related. The kids could "adopt" the older people as foster grandparents, particularly those who don't have grandchildren of their own.

Nothing in the world pleases an older person more than to be called "grandpa" or "grandma" with a feeling of real affection behind it. Wherever programs for foster grandparents exist, those programs have done miracles for the rejuvenation of the aged in their attitudes toward themselves and their ability to function well. Children are wonderfully therapeutic, much better than medicine. Their attitude of love, trust, and affection is something an older person needs very much, and when that older person can return that affection, he or she really begins to feel needed and loved.

Once you get that kind of rejuvenation, once people regain their vigor and their interest in life, the re-emergence of sociability and sexuality is not going to be far behind. Libido—or to put it another way, the "urge"—never dies. Libido in men is almost always present. Libido in women may be dormant for years, but underneath the surface it is there and only needs to be let out. If it is sleeping, it can be awakened—and I've already given you some good examples of that.

When a person who is in an institution regains an interest in life, very often he or she is eager to get out of the institution and go it alone. A big problem with that, however, is money. I'm sure you're all familiar with that problem. The way the rules are now, when older people get married, they lose social security benefits. To me that is an incredibly stupid and short-sighted policy. A couple should be able to live together as man and wife and not be pointed out as people who are living together in sin.

There has been a great deal said about the so-called "living in sin" that is going on these days. Older couples living together without benefit of clergy certainly is common, especially in the resort areas or retirement centers. And as I said, the main reason for it is financial. If that's the reason, and in most cases I'm sure it is, then I see nothing wrong with the practice. However, I deplore the situation that puts people in the spot of having to make that kind of choice.

I'm sure that these men and women who live together without marriage would be perfectly happy being married. No

The Attitudes of Others, and Some Odds and Ends 189

matter how "liberated" they are in their sexual attitudes, the fact that they are living together that way in the face of disapproval of others is bound to make things somewhat difficult for them emotionally. There's nothing I can say to that, except to remind you that you will always be able to find somebody willing to object to almost anything you do because it doesn't jibe with their ideas about the fitness of things.

To paraphrase a well-known statement: you can't satisfy all of the people even some of the time; you can't satisfy even some of the people all of the time; and there's no way on God's green earth you can ever hope to satisfy all of the people all of the time—so why try?

That pretty much covers it. My purpose in this book was to try and convince all of you that sex does not become impossible when you get older, and that sex can be enjoyed at any age, and in any way that is satisfactory to two individuals. It doesn't have to have a pattern, it doesn't have to have a style, and there are no rules. All that is needed is two people who are happy with each other and happy with what they can do together. So allow yourself to have the love, understanding, and companionship you want and deserve. Leave yourself open for a whole new feeling of romance in your life, and a whole new outlook on life.

That new outlook on life is beautifully summed up in an anonymous poem given to me some years ago by a friend:

Youth is not a time of life . . .
It is a state of mind.
Nobody grows old by merely living a number of years.
People grow old by deserting their ideals.

Years wrinkle the skin, but to give up enthusiasm
Wrinkles the soul.

Worry, doubt, self-distrust, fear and despair . . .
These are the long, long years that bow the head
And turn the growing spirit back to dust.

Whether eighty or eighteen, there is in every being's
Heart the love of wonder, the starlike things and
Thoughts, the undaunted challenge of events, the
Unfailing childlike appetite for "what next?" and the
Joy and the game of life.

You are as young as your faith, as old as your doubt,
As young as your self-confidence, as old as your fear,
As young as your hope and as old as your despair.

SEEKING PROFESSIONAL HELP

In no way is this book intended to take the place of counseling and treatment by your family doctor or a qualified therapist. Although I've tried to be as helpful as possible, there are some things that can only be dealt with by actual therapy of some kind.

However, you should be aware that it can be very unwise to just pick the name of a sexual counselor out of the phone book. As in many other fields which are growing in importance, there are many quacks and charlatans posing as professionals. They may do you mental and emotional harm; at any rate, they probably won't do you any good.

The obvious place to begin is your own family doctor, who should be in a better position to help you than anyone else. However, if your doctor doesn't feel qualified, ask for a referral to someone who can help. For those of you without family doctors, here are some organizations which can direct you to reliable professional counselors.

Eastern Association of Sex Therapy
10 E. 88th Street, New York, NY 10028
Contact Don Sloane, M.D.

- American Association of Marriage and Family Counselors
  225 Yale Avenue
  Claremont, California 91711
  Contact Dr. C.R. Fowler

- The American Geriatric Society
  10 Columbus Circle, New York, NY 10019

- The Gerontological Society of Clinical Need
  1 DuPont Circle
  Washington, DC 20036

- Office of Information, National Institute on Aging
  National Institute of Mental Health
  Bethesda, Maryland 20014

You may also contact your local county or state medical society or a nearby school of medicine for the names of qualified people in your area.

SUGGESTIONS FOR FURTHER READING

Although writings on human sexuality can get amazingly complex and technical, there are many really good books written with a general audience in mind. These are some that I've found interesting and helpful. The list is far from complete, and I'm sure you'll find other useful books on your own.

Belliveau, Fred and Richter, Leon. *Understanding Human Sexual Inadequacy,* Little Brown & Co., Boston, 1970. A condensed version of Masters & Johnson's two books, written for the layman and worth reading.

Butler, Robert V. and Lewis, Myrna I. *Sex After 60, A guide for men and women in their later years,* Harper and Row, New York, 1976. Well written and informative.

Comfort, Alex. *The Joy of Sex,* Crown Publishers, Inc., New York, 1972. A bestseller, with voluminous illustrations. Dr. Comfort is one of the outstanding men in the field of geriatrics and sexuality and has written many articles for the profession.

Fromm, Erich. *The Art of Loving,* Harper and Row, New York, 1956.

Hastings, Donald W. *Impotence and Frigidity,* Little Brown & Co., Boston, 1963.

Hastings, Donald W. *A Doctor Speaks on Sexual Expression and Marriage,* Little Brown & Co., Boston, 1966.

Kronhausen, Phyllis & Eberhard. *The Sexually Responsive Woman,* Grove Press, Inc., New York, 1964.

Leif, Harold I. *Medical Aspects of Human Sexuality—750 Questions Answered by 500 Authorities,* Williams and Wilkins Co., Baltimore, Maryland, 1975. A pioneer along with Eric Pfeiffer in the field of geriatrics and sexuality.

McCary, James Leslie Ph.D. *Sexual Myths and Fallacies,* Dan Nostrand Reinhold Co., New York, 1971.

Masters, William H. and Johnson, Virginia E., in association with Robert J. Levin. *The Pleasure Bond—A New Look at Sexuality and Commitment,* Little Brown & Co., Boston, 1970.

J. *The Sensuous Woman,* Dell Publishing Co., New York, 1971.

For those of you who are interested in going beyond the popular treatments of the subject, the following books may be of interest. They are generally intended for professionals engaged in therapy or teaching.

Annon, Jack Ph.D. *Brief Therapy, Vol. I,* Enabling Systems, Inc., Honolulu, Hawaii, 1974.

Brief Therapy, Vol. II—same as above. Highly technical and more for educators, doctors interested in learning sexual therapy.

Butler, Robert N. and Lewis, Myrna I. *Aging and Mental Health,* C.V. Moshy Co., St. Louis, 1973.

Hartman, William E. and Fithian, Marilyn. *Treatment of Sexual Dysfunctions—A Bio-Psycho-Social Approach,* Published by Center for Marital & Sexual Studies, Long Beach, Calif., 1972.

Kaplan, Helen Singer. *The New Sex Therapy,* A Brunner Mazel Publication—published in cooperation with the New York Times Publishing Co.

Kinsey, Alfred C., Pomeroy, Wardell, Martin, and Clyde, E. *Sexual Behavior in the Human Male,* W.B. Saunders & Co., Philadelphia, Pa., 1948.

Kinsey, Alfred C., Pomeroy, Wardell, Clyde, E., and Gelbard. *Sexual Behavior in the Human Female.*

Masters, William H. and Johnson, Virginia E. *Human Sexual Response*, Little Brown & Co., Boston, 1966.
Masters, William H. and Johnson, Virginia E. *Human Sexual Inadequacy*, Little Brown & Co., Boston, 1970.

In addition to the books listed above, much valuable—and highly technical—information is to be found in abstracts from the professional literature. This material can usually be found only in a medical library.

Butler, Robert N. "Medical Advice to the Aging Male"; *Medical Aspects of Human Sex*, September, 1975.
Dean, Stanley R. "Geriatric Sexuality—Normal Needs and Neglected Need"; *Geriatrics*, July, 1974.
Finkle, Alex L. "Sex Life of Aging Person—Pre and Post Prostatectomy effects on Potency." Given at seminar on Sexuality in the Aging—Israel.
Finkle, Alex L. "The Older Patient"; *Medical Aspects of Human Sexuality*, October, 1975. Dr. Finkle, a urologist, has written many papers on sexuality in the male.
Greenblatt, Robert B. "Psychogenic and Endocrine Aspects of Sexual Behavior"; Journal of the American Geriatric Society, 1974.
Greenblatt, Robert B., Sarvey, Edoward. "Sexual Disorders—Hormone Therapy Works"; *Current Prescribing*, 1977. Dr. Greenblatt is probably the foremost authority and pioneer in the field of endocrinology and author of many books and papers.
Pearlman, Carl K. "Frequency of Intercourse in Males at Different Ages"; *Medical Aspects of Human Sexuality*, November, 1972.
Renshaw, Domeena. "Family Physicians—Front Line Therapists"; *The Female Patient*, April, 1977.
Renshaw, Domeena. "A Guide to Sex Counseling"; *The Female Patient*, August, 1977.
Renshaw, Domeena. "How Family Doctors Can Help Patients with Sex Problems"; *Clinical Trends in Family Practice*, November/December, 1976.
Small, Michael P. "Penile Prosthesis for the Management of Impotence"; *Medical Aspects of Human Sexuality*, July, 1976. Describes the two operations in Chapter 12 of this book.

INDEX

Abstinence. *See* Sexuality, and abstinence.
Age, and sexuality. *See* Senility; Sexuality, at advanced age; Sexuality, peak years for.
Alcohol, effect of on sexuality, 51, 54, 115-16, 157
Alcoholism, 51
Aneurysm, 118
Anxiety. *See* Stress.
Apoplexy. *See* Strokes.
Arteriosclerosis, 115, 118
Arthritis, 25, 115, 121, 139

Backache, 115
Birth control. *See* Contraception.
Birth defects, 51
Blood clotting, 48
Blood pressure, 51, 116-17, 119-20
Blood vessel disease, 118

Cancer, 47, 48, 123, 126, 129

Cardiovascular disease, 114
Cauterizing, 35
Cervix, 30, 68
Childbirth, 48
Circumcision, 34, 37, 82
Clitoris, 29, 30, 32, 34, 37, 46, 64, 107, 112, 128, 160
Cocaine, 116
Colostomy surgery, 125-27, 129
Contraception, 92
Counseling. *See* Therapy.
Crosby, Bing, 16

Dating, at advanced age, 178-82
Decongestion, 40, 44
Depression, 20-23, 77-78, 111-12, 146, 172-75, 177
Diabetes, 22, 51, 114, 115, 117
Dilators, 160
Dildos, 151, 160
Drugs, use of, and sexuality, 51, 115, 121, 165, 169-71 (*see also* Alcohol)

Ejaculation. *See* Orgasm, male.
Erection, 24, 36, 37, 41-46, 49, 52, 54, 62, 85, 87, 111-12, 114, 115, 116, 117, 118-19, 137, 143-45, 148-52, 162 *(see also* Impotence)
Estrogen, 29, 46-48, 72
Exercise, 25, 73, 120, 132, 139-40, 178

Fallopian tubes, 38
Fantasies. *See* Sexuality, and fantasies.
Flagyl, 169
Foreplay, 43, 46, 98, 99, 103, 137, 151, 155-56, 160
Frigidity, 64-66, 119, 135, 141, 142; causes of, 66-78, 156, 159, 161; cures for, 71-73, 76-78, 161

Gender, determination of in childbirth, 28-29
Gonorrhea, 17-18, 165, 166-68, 171
Guilt. *See* Sexuality, and guilt.

Hall, Winfield Scott, 81-82
Heart attack, 115, 119-20
Heart disease, 144
Hemophilus vaginalis, 169, 170
Hemorrhoids, 122-23
Heroin, 116
Hormones, artificial, 48, 72; natural, 29, 46-47, 51, 111, 112, 113
Hymen, 34
Hysterectomy, 127-28

Ileostomy surgery, 125, 129
Illness, effects of on sexuality, 21-22, 51, 93, 110-21, 138, 139, 146 *(see also* Diabetes; Heart attack, et al.)
Impotence, 50-51, 65-66, 119, 141, 142, 143; causes of, 51-55, 56, 57, 62, 63, 110-11, 123, 124, 125, 138, 143-45, 146, 150, 151, 156, 173, 181-82; cures for, 55-63, 85, 110-11, 146-51, 153 *(see also* Therapy)
Inhalators, 121
Inhibitions. *See* Sexuality, attitudes about; and inhibitions.
Intimate Life, The (Hall), 81-82

Johnson, Virginia E., 16, 31, 34, 36, 40, 43, 51, 55, 61, 105, 146, 152, 153

Kavanagh, Terence, 120
Kinsey, Alfred C., 16, 17, 31, 105, 184

Labia majora, 29, 33, 35
Labia minora, 29, 33, 35
Leif, Harold I., 31
Libido. *See* Sex drive.
Liver disease, 114
Lubrication, artificial, 111-12; natural, 41, 42, 46, 54, 66, 72, 91, 112, 128, 155, 160, 161, 162
Lung disease, 121

MacArthur, Douglas, 189
Maimonides, 151
Making Love (Raley), 141
Manual stimulation, 43, 48, 64, 162-63 *(see also* Masturbation)
Massage, as therapy, 146-49, 157, 161
Mastectomy, 129

Masters, William H., 16, 31, 34, 36, 40, 43, 51, 55, 61, 105, 146, 152, 153
Masturbation, female, 73, 89-97, 181; male, 51, 60-61, 77-88, 92, 109, 152, 181
Mechanical devices, 151, 160
Menopause, 17, 38, 46, 47, 70-72, 127
Menstruation, 38, 90-91
Morphine, 116
Multiple sclerosis, 51, 115
Myotonia, 40, 41

Narcotics. *See* Drugs.
Neuritis, 115
Nursing homes, 186-88

Oral stimulation, 48, 102-3, 105
Orgasm, female, 23, 24, 40, 43-44, 45, 46, 48-49, 64-65, 66, 68, 76-78, 86, 90-95, 100, 106, 112, 117, 153, 154-58, 159, 160-63; male, 23, 38, 40, 43-44, 45-46, 48-49, 50, 52, 76, 86, 95, 112, 117, 125, 150, 153, 156 (*see also* Premature ejaculation; "Simultaneous" orgasm)
Ovaries, 29, 38, 128
Oviducts. *See* Fallopian tubes.

Pap smears, 48
Parkinson's disease, 176
Penis, 29, 31, 33-34, 36, 37, 41-46, 51, 115, 124, 143, 149, 150, 152, 161
Pfeiffer, Eric, 31
Positions, for sexual intimacy, 118-19, 135-36, 148-50
Pregnancy, 29, 33, 48, 68, 127
Premature ejaculation, 83, 152-53

Priapism, 115
Primary sexual dysfunction, 161-62
Profanity, and sexual intimacy, 100-1
Prostate gland, 25, 38, 42, 52, 123-24
Prostectomy, 52
Psychology Today magazine, 184
Pubic hair, female, 32-33, 35; male, 37-38

Raley, Patricia E., 141
Remarriage, 19, 22-23, 185-86
Retirement, 174-77

Scrotum, 29, 36, 42, 124
Seaman's technique, 152-53
Sedatives. *See* Drugs.
Seminal vesicles, 38, 42
Senile vaginitis, 72, 95, 115
Senility, 173-75
Sex drive, female, 17-24, 61, 68, 69-75, 117; male, 17-21, 50, 52, 56-58, 69-70
Sex organs, female, 28-35, 36, 37, 38, 39-49, 54, 64, 68, 91-95, 107, 112, 115, 117, 128, 146, 149, 150, 152, 155, 160, 161, 162, 169; male, 28-31, 33-34, 36-38, 39-49, 51, 52, 79, 115, 117, 124, 146, 149, 150, 152, 161; size of, female, 33-34; size of, male, 36-37
Sexual dysfunction. *See* Frigidity; Impotence; Primary sexual dysfunction.
Sexual intercourse without penetration, 23-24
Sexuality, and abstinence, 16-20, 46, 181-82, 184; at advanced age, 15-27, 35, 45, 46, 47,

Sexuality *(Cont.)*
  48-49, 55-61, 68-71, 72, 75, 80-81, 87-88, 93, 95-97, 105, 108, 114, 152, 153, 162, 164, 173-82, 184-85, 187-88;
  attitudes about, 15-19, 25-27, 29, 31, 36-37, 50-52, 55, 58-61, 64-66, 68-71, 73, 79-84, 89-94, 127-28, 134-35, 161, 183-88; disinterest in, 133-38; and fantasies, 86, 94, 107-8; fears about, 67, 110-11, 121, 138, 143, 145-46, 150, 159, 162, 173, 181-82; and guilt, 83-84, 85, 90-95, 96, 104; and inhibitions, 78, 85, 116, 138, 155, 181 *(see also* Sexuality, attitudes about); peak years for, 16, 20-21, 41, 65-66, 69, 75, 80
Sexually transmitted disease. *See* Venereal disease.
"Sexual revolution," 26-27, 183
Sexual satisfaction, achieving, 15, 19, 24, 32, 98-109, 131-42 *(see also* Stimulation)
Silicone implants, 129, 151-52
"Simultaneous" orgasm, 156-57
Spastic conditions, 121
"Spectatoring," 146
"Squeeze" technique, 152-53
Stimulation, sexual, 23-24, 32, 37, 40-46, 48-49, 53, 54, 66, 73, 78, 86, 91, 93, 94, 96, 111, 112-13, 138, 146-50, 151, 157, 160-61 *(see also* Erection; Lubrication)
Stress, mental, effects of on sexuality, 52, 54, 80-81, 87, 146, 157-59, 173
Strokes (apoplexy), 23, 25, 115, 118-19
Sulcus, 37

Surgery, effects of on sexuality, 122-30
Syphilis, 165-69, 171

Tension. *See* Stress.
Testicles, 29, 36, 41, 42, 45
Testosterone, 29
Therapy, for sexual dysfunction, arranging for, 191-92; physical, 138, 139-40, 141, 146-49, 160-61; psychological, 81, 84, 112, 138, 139, 140-42, 144-45, 159, 176 *(see also* Frigidity; Impotence, cures for)
Tranquilizers. *See* Drugs.
Trichomonas vaginalis, 169

Urethra, 30, 35, 38, 124, 166
Urethral meatus, 34, 37, 42
Urination, 30, 31, 34, 37, 42, 93, 124
Uterus, 38, 47, 49, 128

Vagina, 29, 30, 35, 41-44, 46-49, 54, 67, 68, 72, 91, 92, 112, 115, 128, 149, 150, 152, 155, 160, 161, 162, 169
Vaginismus, 67, 115, 160, 161
Vas deferens, 38
Vasocongestion, 40, 41, 43, 112
Venereal disease, 17-18, 164-71; cures for, 167-68, 169; preventives against, 168, 170; symptoms of, 166-67, 169-70
Vigor, sexual. *See* Sexuality, peak years for.
Virginity, 34, 68
Vulva, 33

Wet dreams, 85
Women's movement, 27

Yeast infections, 165, 169, 170